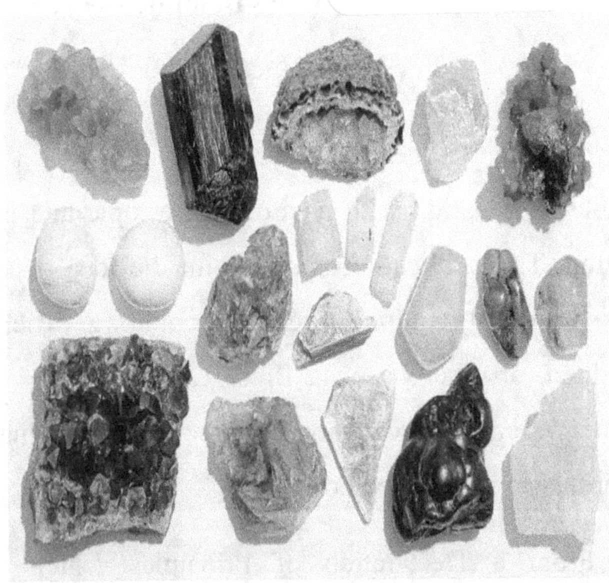

CRYSTALS FOR BEGINNERS

The Complete Guide

To

Discover The Healing Power Of Crystals

TABLE OF CONTENTS

INTRODUCTION

rystals are stunning gems that are traditionally been used for healing and divination for centuries. It's been found to be effective to help alleviate stress and heal the body.

It's no surprise that some people, including famous and wealthy ones, have opted for crystal healing, a non-invasive therapy that is based on those sparkly, transparent stones due to their perceived curative and healthy properties.

Crystals can magically enable and enhance every part of your daily life. Everything from easy relaxation techniques to finding past lives and healing health problems.

A kind of crystal is quartz - considered by many to possess. The operation is again and associated with the utilization in metaphysics and chakra healing

Quartz are also patented with the healing and magical property use in electronic equipment and science.

Quartz may come in various shape, sizes, and signs. The quartz crystals used by people are walnut, gemini, and tiger eye.

Crystals can help you in clearing the mind from any anxiety. Some take a crystal while driving so as to maintain safe.

Crystals have a power to safeguard your loved ones and friends, keep the evil away, to and draw decent luck, riches

Crystals do not only promotes your self-esteem but they also boost your clarity of intention.

The tiger eye crystal for instance, is highly valued and respected by people who wear it for its benefits and curative power. It drives your will towards success and encourages your enthusiasm.

Many individuals no matter the sex or age like to use crystals for multiple reasons. Africans, by way of example, utilize magic to be warded off by crystals.

They believe that curses exist frequently so it's essential to walk around as security with the tiger's eye crystals.

Crystals are powerful energy sources that can be utilized to promote healing. Healing with crystals works with psychological, spiritual and physical issues by taking away the dis-ease at ease on your own, and making you.

Choosing a crystal for a specific reason focus on then and that motive allow your intuition to decide on the proper crystals. There are a lots and lots of crystals to choose from for any particular reason.

There are the diamond, amazonite, aventurine, gold, peridot, emerald, green tourmaline, and many more. Concentrate on the purpose and motives and allow your intuition guide you to the ideal crystal.

Crystals can subtly assist to bring the energy vibrations into a lively and healthy balance within your body and aura and also transmit energy vibrations.

Crystals can likewise be aligned with our energy and can also act on our energy fields. They also assist in creating scenarios in lives that leads us in directions that enable healing and positive growth.

Crystals can be used in many ways - the hottest is to

wear your crystal. Your crystal can be charged to entice vibrations and energies and protect you.

Crystals may also be put in your surroundings or house for exactly the same purpose- this is particularly effective when following the principles of Feng Shui.

Crystals are also popularly known as pendulums, also used for divination to answer easy yes/no questions.

Crystals can also be used in healing, by placing crystals to the energy centers (chakras) of the body to strengthen and rebalance the circulation of the body's own ability to heal.

This beginner's manual will help you learn more about clearing, orientation, recovery, cleansing, maintenance and crystal formation.

A crystal can be the finest multi-purpose tool for your own personal development!

Happy Reading!

CHAPTER 1
WHAT ARE CRYSTALS?

The Crystals or gemstones are distinctive sorts of rocks with properties or naturally occurring minerals. The difference between a crystal and a stone is in its own atom and molecular construction.

Crystals are usually constructed of a single or a couple of kinds of atoms that form atom patterns that were replicating.

A unique property of crystals is that they form over time. The process of growth of crystals is called crystallization.

Because of their structure, crystals are able to store, receive, and transmit electricity. This energy may be used for healing in so called 'crystal therapy' - a frequent alternative practice of recovery.

Crystal meditation is a practice of combining the energy of crystals or placing them on chakras with meditation practices that are distinct.

Crystals are 'friends' in such a way that they affect the energy of the location if used as objects and have around and garnish.

They are also able to improve energy area and of people wearing them. Energies are emitted by gemstones of unique types and ought to be used in line with their vibration and their possessions.

For proper use of gemstones for energy and healing work, it is required to learn certain knowledge and practices of working with crystals, power and intention.

Very simple to learn and things are how to clean, charge and program your own crystals.

Crystal can be strong tool for healing an individual's psychological, spiritual and vitality ailments that are closely connected to all physical symptoms we call illnesses.

Crystals have healing powers.

Crystals are energy in solid form as is everything on the planet and in the world. Why are crystals so helpful to us? Well, our body is made from electromagnetic systems, also referred to as power systems.

Nature has created crystals to be perfect conductors, they interact perfectly with our system.

Crystals have been found to take vibration which triggers the energy centers within our system.

Crystals in Egypt were utilized in temples to connect more deeply with the infinite, to cure their own bodies and to help individuals transform emotions.

Crystals are used by cultures throughout the world for centuries for balancing and healing the human race.

Each crystal has a distinctive vibration and we can use them to areas of the body, or soother organs, or activate.

You can learn how to use them easily with a bit of help from the right brain. The brain is the one that works everything out, the brain is the intuitive one, the one that gets hunches. Relax and let us find out a little more about our healing crystals.

Some of the most common but very successful and robust healing stones for beginners are:

Red Jasper - For strengthening the fundamental energy of an individual, ideal for root chakra (1st).

Tiger's eye - Builds self-esteem and raises faith. Works on sacral chakra (2nd).

Citrine - Amplifies energy that is life-force, brings positive and light vibrations trough solar plexus chakra (3rd).

Aventurine or Rose Quartz - Best for opening the heart, bringing stability love and connection. Usual use is on the heart chakra (4th).

Calcedone - opens and strengthens the center for self-expressing and willpower. It's usage is situated on the throat chakra (5th).

Amethyst – This crystal strengthens the link to spiritual energy and raises intuition, for use on the third eye chakra (6th)

Clear Quartz - purest crystal energy for balancing and amplifying work of all chakras and energy systems. You may use it to the crown chakra (7th).

Some crystals are powerful than other people, you will know which ones are right for you, when you use the exercise.

Crystals are presents from the ground, how amazing our curing powers are also and the more people use them the more we discover these crystals are.

The role of using healing crystals is to reestablish the balance of energies and also to return the physical creature being to a wholesome state.

Crystals and Gemstones are one of the most amazing, mysterious and profound "energy medicine" tools, that are used for centuries in all religions, cultures, and empires.

With the need for non-physical healing and physical healing combined, many people are discovering the power of healing crystals.

Crystals are used in spiritual and meditation ceremonies and are also laid on the body during bodywork or massages when an individual is bathing, drinking or resting inside water.

They bring awe-inspiring benefits to the healing centers. Crystals, gemstones and minerals can be powerful tools in teaching us how to heal ourselves. Crystals are found in all shapes, sizes, colors and composition.

Crystals can be selected by their related curative properties or they can be chosen by the color that's associated with the chakra regulating the particular disorder, disease, disorder or area of your life that needs healing or balancing.

Crystals of various color's help in the healing process by changing the state of mind and producing tranquil emotions.

The feelings and intuitions that you get may be subtle, it won't be like an "explosion of fireworks", but when you start trusting yourself and your feelings, your inner guidance will get stronger, and you will subconsciously know/feel what to do or which healing crystals to use at which days.

You will learn about healing crystals in the next chapters by paying attention to how they make you feel.

The travel you start to travel with healing crystals will change your life forever and you'll grow to appreciate them as they enhance your world and help you on all levels.

Some of the different kinds of Healing crystals to try could include:

Agates - aid the wearer feel protected and are effective for children. They also help to center your thoughts and feelings

Amethyst - effective for stress or melancholy and headaches/migraines, bring serenity and calm during meditation, is known as a Master Healing Stone

Chakras - gain mind soul and leads to a greater sense of stability and inner equilibrium

Rose Quartz - for emotional healing, love, beauty, peacefulness, forgiving, self-indulgent & self esteem

Crystals have been an important part of this healing world has ever walked upon this ground. We can all benefit from the energy of crystals.

The Functions and Effects of Crystal

Crystal is a very common sort of jewelry material, as we know this. It's adored by many people because of its bright colors and clearness.

But, there are five main effects and functions of crystal that are confirmed by the lengthy time study of scholars and experts. The functions are alter, storage, move, focus and amplify.

Focus

In ancient times, human beings had found the refraction of light of crystal and the focus function of clear.

With this attribute, it can be made to convex, concave and so on. The crystal that's strong, highly parallel and exact can be applied to eye surgery. Giant ones may be used to destroy incoming missiles and so on.

Storage

The information will be recorded by crystal, which is

just, when a message passes through the crystal. So do the spectrometer lens, prism, etc. in contemporary times.

Piezoelectric crystal will take on positive and negative charges that are the computer binary 1 and 0.

Yes, this is actually the basis of the computer. Until today, memory's storage capacity is amazing. You are able to input of the info in the Encyclopedia.

Transfer

The transmissions of information of appliances also rely on in the processor, because the crystal oscillation frequency is stable; and there's rarely an error to pass tokens.

As the crystal oscillator chip is very precise and regular, in addition to be utilized as the time control of electronic form, it may also be utilized to make the computer function calculation as well as the transmission of message that was huge.

Transform

Electricity can be converted by crystal to other sources, like converting the energy into sound energy, heat, light and energy;.

The collector chip will be needed by turning power. Sound, light, power, heat are all energies. They're immortal, just being changed to another form or state; along with the crystal is your best matchmaker.

Amplify

Crystal make them remain in the same frequency and can enhance the energy passing through.

For example, when using a megaphone, the current moves through the quartz and transforms into noise energy (energy conversion), and then enriches the voices (energy expansion), and the tone will not be changed (frequency invariability).

Sign can be expanded by crystal like crystals convert them into noise, which can be noticed by people's ears, and in the radio is going to obtain the ratio tide in the atmosphere.

Well, if we don't discover, we'll never know that crystal has so many functions. In a word, crystal is a very lovely kind of jewelry in addition to a powerful "weapon".

CHAPTER 2
THE EXISTENCE OF
CRYSTALS

To most of us, who've spent our lives grounded in the physical, which we referred to as "fact", the concept of crystal recovery has made its way to irrational superstition and the new age.

It's as if many of us are asking, how in the world can a rock be anything more than a rock less energy or help us cure? How do minerals, rocks and metals do anything but just sit there?

To answer this question, we must venture beyond the physical existence which we currently think is "all there is" to this reality we're living in.

Issue has been seen as the foundation of reality. To put it differently, physicality is the evaluation most of us use to ascertain what is "real" from what's "not real".

But matter is not the middle of fact as we know it. Instead, it is only a tiny aspect of boundless energy within the world.

You might think of physical reality such as the universe, much like skin's thin membrane.

A layer of skin, covering an hidden substructure of additional vast measurements where energy is expressed differently because it vibrates at different frequencies depending on the size it exists in.

Every object that is single whether it's alive or not living is present within this physical level, but also from the multitude of dimensions that are energetic outside physicality.

All you find in this world is multidimensional in nature. Your full bodily system is nothing more than energy that shows up in a variety of patterns and densities. The same goes for what we believe to be "inanimate structures" like rocks.

When patterns of energy work together in a non-resistant and cohesive way we experience what we call health.

A great number of things can disrupts All these patterns of energy. We encounter a country of dis-ease when this occurs.

This leads to bad health. This immune, discordant energy patterning is responsible for every negative symptom we encounter in our physical out of, everything from a headache to cancer.

Everything we believe is solid and "actual" is only emerging real to us due to our physical senses, but our bodily senses do merely interpreting energy for a scent or as a sight or a taste of a feel.

It's our senses which convert what is for want of a better word an energetic, holographic reality to the static reality we call bodily.

It is our senses that tell us we are "different" from our environment. At our most fundamental level, we are not participating in this vast field, we're also made of the field. We're one with each inanimate and animate thing we all see.

Our real lives are different expressions of the exact same power that makes up "all that's" across every world and in each dimension. The amplitude and frequency (that which we often call vibration) where this energy expresses itself, is what determines if energy becomes a rock or a person in physical measurement.

Crystals and what we predict as gemstones, possess a vibration which is free of patterns that are resistant.

They are among a number of those constructions from the measurement which have the balanced, intentional, strong and cohesive frequencies.

Their un-changing physical construction is a manifestation of the truth that their energetic patterns of strength and balance and cohesiveness are incorruptible.

In the physical measurement when you get a crystal it might look as if you are not doing more than looking or touching another, physical thing.

But in the other dimensions in which both you and the stone exist, you are "entraining" energetically with this stone.

Changes are subsequently caused by this entrainment to your structure and psychology on the physical dimension. The governing law of each dimension within the universe is that of "oneness". In bodily life, we've
18

begun to call this the "Law of Attraction".

Accordingly, so as to share the identical space with a different "form", you must be moving in precisely the exact same level since it is vibrating. Health is the natural state of any form within the universe.

Therefore the inclination and trend of anything within the world is that of cohesiveness equilibrium and simplicity.

This means that the natural development of vibration would be to entrain and resonate in the path of health.

Because of this, when you talk about the distance that a crystal (or bead) which has a resistance free vibration, then rather than the vibration of the crystal embracing a non-cohesive pattern, your electricity will entrain with all the energy of this crystal and embrace it's cohesive pattern.

This causes one to no longer produce the routine of dis-ease inside your energetic substructures and therefore the physical manifestation of that dis-eased energy is no longer being maintained and the bodily symptom disappears.

As a result of this effect, crystals and diamonds are proficient at bringing us back into a state of stability and health.

Anything having an inherent energetic pattern of non-resistance can behave by offering a vibration which we could use to re-tune ourselves into a healthy vibration.

This is really happening on the energetic levels of substructure if you listen to a tune which makes you feel good, or spend some time near a person that makes you feel good, or take a homeopathic treatment.

Every crystal or gemstone resonates with a slightly different pattern energetically, and therefore looks different in the physical in terms of things like chemical geometry, color, composition, structure, and texture. Because of this, each one lends itself to patterns which live within our bodily systems.

For example, with rose quartz would be to expose the lively patterns active in our physical and metaphoric heart to align themselves with health and embrace a much more immunity free pattern.

Therefore, when we entrain with increased quarts,

unresolved heart problems will dissipate, allowing us to let go of what's distorting our energies which identify with the center.

Gemstones and crystals grow profound within in the earth's crust over countless years at heat and very substantial pressures.

This gives them a place among the objects on earth with the energy that is . They're capable of reflecting energy, including, casting, emanating, refracting, and receiving.

Crystals have a consistent arrangement of atoms. From the stone referred to as "quartz", these atoms vibrate at a stable and measurable frequency, due to this, quartz an excellent receiver and emitter of energy that is stored. As a result of this, quartz is used in watches, radios and numerous electronic technologies.

Just like power, thought is a type of energy which could be given leadership by that which we call "intention". Crystals can be programmed without power, utilizing only thoughts as the informational energy.

Quartz is also known as a piezoelectric material i.e.

something which produces an electric charge when a stress is applied.

When conductive substance is placed under mechanical pressure, a shifting of the negative and positive charge centers in the substance takes place, which then ends in an external electrical field.

The stress can also be caused by twisting or hitting the material without fracturing it in other to deform its crystal lattice.

This effect likewise works in the other way, with the material when a small electrical current is applied deforming.

While the argument rages back and forth as to if the piezoelectric effect contributes to the human-crystal recovery relationship or not, the fact that crystals are so responsive to electro-magnetic fields has severe consequences.

It has implications since our bodies are composed of and constantly emanating electro-magnetic areas and crystals and gemstones respond to this power that is generating and coursing through our bodies.

Another interesting finding is that quartz is composed of silicon and oxygen (SiO2), a mixture known to Geologists of minerals as the building block. Our world consists of minerals comprising silicon and oxygen

Silicon is a significant constituent of our bodies. Some of the science oriented people have speculated that the transport of energy in the natural crystal into the silicon within our bodies might have something to do with the bodily healing effect caused by exposure to crystals.

Crystals and Gemstones are just one of the most powerful tools available to people in the physical dimension of presence.

It's a tool all people have employed subconsciously at one time or another. Often it's an interaction that occurs by our attention being drawn to a specific stone.

We think it is "pretty" although we do not understand why we like it so much we feel compelled to pick it up and keep it in our pocket. We've got no idea why this urge was believed by us and we don't have any conscious awareness of what is behind our impulse to pick this up.

We have no idea that our lively substructure is calling us towards the particular vibration of that rock in order to entrain together and proceed towards a more cohesive healthy pattern compared to the one we are currently maintaining in ourselves.

Like all tools, the key to utilization is to learn how to consciously implement the tool.

If this type of fore mentioned situation could cross from a subconscious compulsion to a conscious process of looking for a particular crystal or gemstone based on understanding of the benefit of using it, the person's receptivity will be that the effects of the entrainment would be a hundred fold.

If we recognized that the quality of gemstone and every crystal impacts our own fields, we'd see that they create an electro- chemical response inside our body and psychology that would allow us to utilize them since the tools that they are.

They could be used by us on a daily basis to promote evolution, awareness, growth and wellbeing in the multidimensional and ourselves lives we live.

CHAPTER 3
THE SPIRITUAL WORLD OF CRYSTALS

For shamans, ages and crystal healers have been familiar with the crystals' capacity to concentrate sound and light vibrations into a mixed ray for purposes of healing.

They have been used to realign energies by helping to get to the root of the issue, and dissolve dis-ease.

Reverence and application of crystals goes back into the dawning of culture. Crystals are linked with specific areas of the body and its organs for thousands of years and lots of these connections come in conventional Eastern and Western Astrology.

And is recorded by the Ayurvedic of india, Traditional chinese medicine proves healing with crystals, which appear in ancient text formulas over 5,000 years old, now widely used in modern medical prescriptions.

The Bible describes crystals over 200 times as crystalline structures found in Chinese tombs of rulers and the ancient Egyptian, and at the ruins of Babylonia, lots of the early civilizations of the Earth (American Indian, Mayan, Aztec, African, Celtic) employed stone crystals at sacred ceremonies.

Individuals have always been drawn to Crystals, primarily because of their visual appeal, exquisite purity, fantastic interplay of colors and also "crystal-clear" transparency.

Crystals, semi-precious and precious stones, but have other outstanding features, making them very much convenient to be used as tools in various metaphysical, spiritual, and therapeutic practices.

The spiritual science believes as living beings which are at the simple level of development of consciousness crystals and all the members of the mineral kingdom.

This is compared to the belief that is widely spread based on todays' science parameters in which crystals are not categorized as living entities.

Various vibrations crystals are capable of collecting

energy. What's more, they can amplify the energy and bring it back to us and our environment through vibration and resonance.

Their assistance can be priceless, provided that we handle them. After we've mastered the art of communication with our crystals, they are going to reveal to us more - their hidden virtues and qualities.

It's believed that the religious basis of coping with crystals originates from Atlantis, where a potent technology for obtaining crystals synthetically had been invented, enabling production of crystals of extended proportions for use for different purposes.

Amid the number of crystals that are available, it might be hard for all of us to choose the ideal crystal.

There are a number of essential points of picking crystals which should be considered before creating our thoughts, for example visual appeal, intuitive appeal and attraction at mental level, and crystal's practical values.

Once the crystal has been chosen for instance, by using the help of one of the four elements (fire, water, earth and air) we could control and application it.

By charging, we associate it with all the types and qualities of energy we would like to place within our crystal.

By programming, we augment our selected intentions, feelings, and thoughts to the crystal energy routine, and our crystal will enhance and irradiate them back to us.

The color of crystals can be a fantastic indication as to what sort of metaphysical clinic or therapeutic practice their specific energies are acceptable for.

For example, white or purple crystals open the doorway of perception; bring unity. Red crystals are symbols of life, vitality, power. Energies are moved by them, they worm up.

Life is encouraged by orange crystals energy, self-control and regulate the performance of the glands.

Yellow crystals influence the operation of gallbladder, kidneys, the liver, and spleen and also assist indigestion.

They release subconscious fears, balance is promoted by and. green crystals represent the color of harmony, health, love and creativity.

They help to regulate the blood pressure, heart disorders, stimulate love and calm the nerves.

Ultimately, it's important to remember that crystals been occupying the omnipresent cosmic love, spreading their continuous vibrations of energy and amplifying it.

They've been supporting God's production, by outpouring their spirituality and love to the world, transmitting the Sun's light, love, and warmth, and along with it, their structural stability. Because of this, it is comforting to know they can be our devoted friends, teachers and advisers.

Crystals As Alchemy For the Body and Soul

The earth consciousness supports humanity's awakening to re-discovery of ancient healing arts, such as crystals.

Crystals are universal energies which allow you to get these individual energies for integration and healing.

Each crystal comprises their own "character" can also

be utilized in unique techniques to assist comprehension of the nature of presence on the Earth plane. Crystals are nature's gift to man and are located in all shapes, sizes, colors, and composition.

They each have a distinctive vibrational resonance due to their varying mineral materials, their inherent geometry, and the color frequency they exude; hence may be powerful recovery tools.

Crystal healing is a method whereby gemstones are put on the body, utilized as reflex tools to stimulate points on the feet, worn, or could be placed around one's home to boost feng shui energy.

Exactly the identical color crystals can be placed on the other corresponding one to enhance stream of energy or you can only meditate by holding the crystal into the third eye (6th chakra) to obtain messages or energy.

They heal on physical, mental, emotional, and spiritual levels, helping to guide the flow of energy to a particular portion of the body, restore balance, and finally cleanse by releasing and releasing blocked energy.

The vibrational of the body energy is a complex electromagnetic system which the crystals are capable of interacting with because they're nature's best electromagnetic conductors.

Crystals work through resonance and have been found to carry vibrations which trigger specific energy centers, favorably affecting our body system.

Some crystals also contain minerals known for their curative abilities used in medical practices.

They're piezoelectric, meaning light and power is produced by compression and can produce sound waves that.

Choosing a crystal to utilize can be as straightforward as following your instinct about that captures the gist of the energy you're drawn to, or you can reference crystal recovery indicators to help you associate symptoms with relevant crystals.

These beings that are powerful are sacred tools to encourage us on our individual journeys and serve as route to harmonious balance, higher consciousness, personal evolution, well-being, subconscious unveiling, and healing support.

Crystal healing is clarity that is celestial to be activated by an alchemical process that blends crystal energy with our core vibration.

CHAPTER 4
THE MYRIAD COLORS OF CRYSTALS

Though it is not a documented fact, it's quite safe to say there are so many crystals as there are colors that represent them.

The lore of every form of crystal and its own inherent healing assets continues to be passed down from generation to generation, and comparable to Chinese drug stores which specialize in herbal mixtures for remedies of all types of ailments, crystals have distinct yet delicate healing and enhancement facilities.

Wondering which crystal to choose for a particular need? Below is a list of several of the Most Popular crystals, and the main purposes for their application:

Amethyst - (purple/violet) - That the immune and endocrine system strengthens, and it is also a blood cleanser and energizer.

In addition, it enhances channeling and psychic

abilities and helps alleviate mental distress and ailments. The Amethyst crystal is quite calming, and therefore it's an excellent crystal to use for meditation.

Aventurine - (sea-green/forest-green) - The venturine crystal is thought to purify the "three bodies" - the psychological, emotional, and etheric, or "aural" body that extends only outside what appears to be the "advantages" of your physical body.

It thereby encourages freedom and also aids in releasing fear and anxiety.

Carnelian - (bright orange) - Alleviates and memory sorrow and grief enhances. Creativity and courage also increases while lessening fear, jealousy, and anger.

Many men and women carry the Carnelian crystal for protection and decent luck. Hint: It can assist you in finding the proper mate!

Fluorite - (milky white, clear, mild green, slate gray) - The properties of this Fluorite crystal are just what you most likely already picture: they reinforce your bones and teeth!

They are known as the "health" crystals, as they are

also quite beneficial for keeping the blood vessels along with the spleen apparent of any toxins.

Fluorite crystals ground and "slough off" surplus energy, so they are also excellent for the progress of their brain, concentration, and meditation.

For those of you who are interested in communication, fluorite will also keep you strong and healthy while connecting with inter-dimensional beings.

Clear Quartz - (white, clear) - The clear quartz crystal might be the most popular simply. This crystal enhances and activates both the pineal and pituitary glands, which regulate growth, therefore this crystal is recommended for children and teens, in particular.

These crystals also serve as Great psychological "balancers" while amplifying the thought process, making clairvoyance which much easier.

Hang these crystals facing a window to allow the full spectrum of energy activate your entire degrees of consciousness, particularly when you're feeling down - these crystals are pros at dispelling negative energy.

Lapis - (blue or topaz) - This crystal is very effective

for the internal organs: utilize this crystal if you suffer from acid reflux, migraines, or other digestive troubles, or bloating. Additionally, it also assist in spiritual development.

Hematite - (silver gray/dark Grey) - Hematite has a very positive influence on the smooth flow of the bloodstream.

It also removes toxins from and triggers spleen activity, which filters blood and regulates the red blood cells with the white blood cells.

Hematite can also be used to relieve anxiety and strengthen the physical body; it's unique energizing properties, and in addition, it enhances personal magnetism, which of course boosts confidence, courage, and all those great things!

Rose Quartz - (pink/rose) - It is believed to increase fertility and ease psychological and sexual imbalances, crystal is found close to the mind. Obviously, this frees away stored-up anger.

Take a hot temper, or a buddy who flares a bit too much? Get a Rose Quartz crystal! "Everything sweet" is the best description for this crystal, which also promotes enlightenment, compassion, and love. Nobody should be without it!

Jasper - (/spotted/ light Brown/flecked) - This crystal emits tremendous mental and emotional recovery, and it promotes stability and equilibrium. It also alleviates anxieties, hopes, and shows ideas. It enhances visualization, so take note as you meditate.

Moonstone - (Bluish-green/Cream) - This crystal is connected with protection and love, and it also drums up additional psychic and intuition skills.

Obsidian - (black/gray) - This crystal is a favorite because it brings a feeling of purity and serenity to those who carry, wear, or use it for healing purposes.

It brings both positive and negative emotions to the surface, offering balance in times of transition and change.

Sodalite - (smoky blue/clear, Dark blue) - This stunning crystal is also an inner-organ healer; it favorably affects the endocrine and endocrine system.

Also, it is said to remove fear and also has a method

of balancing the male/female, or yin/yang polarities in those who believe in need of "centering." It also is great for communication and creative expression.

Tiger Eye - (brown/striped/tan/yellow) - This is just another crystal many men and women carry around for health purposes: Tiger Eye crystals cover nearly everything: the spleen, intestines, pancreas, and the colon.

It is extremely grounding and centering. Have a stubborn friend? Slip one of these into his or her pocket as a token of love. They'll direct having a sudden clear sense of insight and perception to yo

CHAPTER 5
COLOR CRYSTAL DIVINATION FOR TAPPING INTO THE ENERGY OF THE EARTH

Crystals have been used as a tool for divination as far back as the times of the Druids. Many believe crystals contain the earth's energy and, by tapping into the power of crystals, an individual can experience healing shifts and awareness.

In crystal divination, crystals may be used change or to affect one's energy, and in many cases, color crystal divination can alter the results of one's present or future scenarios.

Crystals come in various sizes, shapes and colors. It's believed that these differing variables determine the unique vibration of energy of each crystal.

For all, this energy could be felt or obtained through mediation or shifts in consciousness. In crystal readings, it's believed that one can tap by working with particular colors.

Color crystal divination isn't unlike candle divination. Each crystal has its own meaning. The most important element in crystal divination is choosing.

In crystal divination, it's always important to utilize colors which have relationships. For instance, if you are experiencing difficulties with your connection, you'd work with reddish colored crystals like agate or garnet.

Below I've listed the main colors utilized in color candle divination. When working with color crystal divination, it is always important to make sure you clean your crystals under running water until you work with them.

Not only does this cleanse any energy, it also helps the flow and release of the crystal vibrations.

White: New beginnings, partnerships, and jobs. White crystals are effective at encouraging change or assisting you to identify decisions that are important.

White is the color of purity and can also assist with emotional or religious cleansing.

Black: Endings and grief. Black is the color of letting go. It is a color that encourages acceptance and internal transformation. Black may also be a color of conclusion or finished company.

Brown: Brown is the color of earth. Owing to its institution to earth, brown relates to all things that happen within the world: money, home, and security.

Pink: Friendships, family reconciliations. Pink is the color of sensitivity, patience and compassion. In crystal divination, pink can help to bring opposites together and promotes peace and neutrality.

Red: Fireplace Love, and Romance. Red may also be utilized for the readiness and courage to face One's anxieties.

In crystal divination, reddish can be used to assist themselves are asserted by one in a manner.

Orange: Happiness, Equilibrium and independence. In crystal divination that is color, orange can help promote balance and harmony. Additionally, it can help with self-esteem and self-confidence.

Yellow: Communication, self-expression and clarity.

Yellow relates to the usage of the logic and reasoning abilities of one.

Green: bitterness and feelings. In The color green, Color crystal divination helps you get in touch with your feelings that are true.

Blue: Healing and equality. Blue may be used for matters where there has been some injustice.

Blue represents fairness and equilibrium. In addition, it can be used for healing the physical body.

Purple: Psychic Intuition, Psychic development and intellect. Purple may also help one get in touch with the unconscious and help one in things that concern sleep or dreams

CHAPTER 6
USING THE LAW AND QUARTZ CRYSTALS OF ATTRACTION

Countless individuals in the world are now aware about the Law of Attraction.

In this chapter, I will review the basic principles of the Law of Attraction and how you can achieve powerful results in your life using quartz crystals to boost the process of reflection guaranteed with the Law of Attraction.

Your Thoughts Determine Your Life

In a nutshell, the Law of Attraction claims that the reality we experience in our lives-our degree of success, happiness, love, and abundance-is determined by feelings and our thoughts.

Anything you focus on many intently on your thoughts, whether good or bad, more of that comes.

Manifestation occurs in 3 measures. These steps are utilized in several commercially accessible coaching systems and other programs for self-improvement, wealth, and success:

STEP 1: Your desire takes your aims, shape on dreams, and goals that are particular.

STEP 2: The world hears your calls and they hold your desire for you.

STEP 3: You align using a higher frequency that permits the manifestation.

In this chapter, we will take a closer look at these steps, you will learn how you to use quartz crystals to boost the manifestation process.

Putting the 3 Manifestation Steps into Action

STEP 1 Your desire. We've got so many wishes that we constantly act out and they need to be tuned in a particular manner; otherwise they are arbitrary and lack focused energy.

Getting fulfillment of your wants is like searching on Google: To receive the returns which you want, you need to make your request unique and clear. If you conduct a search for "house" you'll likely get 1.3 billion hits!

If you search for "house, 2 Tales, green, Maui, under $500,000" you'll become far fewer hits as you narrow in on your goal. The ideas and requests that you send out to the world need to be exceptionally focused and unique.

Visualize your desired outcome, its exact attributes, and when you intend to achieve it. In your head, ardently look for the end result of attaining your goal, possibly far better than you can envision it.

STEP 2: Trust the world has heard your request. This step happens without your awareness, therefore you don't have to bother yourself. Be rest assured that the world will do its own part to receive and hold as chances your stated goals.

STEP 3: Align with a higher frequency. The next step is that the work you've got to do in order to achieve what you want.

To repeat, whatever you concentrate on you will attract to your life. If you concentrate on a problem that's extremely vexing to you personally, this is what you're aligning yourself with-with the unwanted energies of the problem, not with what you want rather than the problem.

Inevitably, we are given by problems bad feelings. In the event you choose to concentrate on these feelings that are terrible, you are giving them more energy.

Luckily, it is possible to consciously choose to shift your focus to the solution to everything you wish to bring to your own life rather than the problem.

If you do immediately notice your internal state shifts to more positive emotions. Your mind opens to some stream of solutions and ideas.

You will shortly feel you are mastering the problem instead of being dis-empowered by it.

It's vital to make a practice of continuously tracking your state and readjusting your ideas and feelings so they are aligned with your aims, rather than in resistance. Thoughts oppose and negate your true needs.

Positive feelings and thoughts strengthens your true desires. If you embrace this observation and adjust your habit, instantly substituting your positive thoughts for the negative ones, you'll just discover yourself feeling good all the time and ready to proceed with resilience beyond all obstacles.

In addition to their beauty, crystals possess metaphysical qualities which you may use in several fabulous ways to enhance your life.

The most enticing of these attributes is that the ability of crystals to keep info for you and function as a focal point for your own intentions and prayers.

There is a crystal like a computer chip in which you are able to save information. And in fact a computer processor is made out of silicon, quartz crystals' basic ingredient.

Crystals can assist you with measures of aligning yourself consciously with your dreams and desires by aligning you with the flow toward your objectives, upping your energy frequency, and helping you anchor yourself is a favorable inner state.

The Metaphysical Properties and Uses of

Quartz Crystals

Quartz is the most common of all crystals, located all around the world. It is made up of carbon dioxide, which is among the compounds of the Earth's crust. It grows in cluster and is frequently found in conjunction with other minerals too.

Crystal quartz is very clear and Translucent in its appearance and therefore it is the manifestation of clarity and lighting. It signifies our increasing our consciousness toward higher degrees and striving for perfection in our internal growth.

Astrologically crystal quartz reflects the properties of the Sun (mild) and Saturn (crystallization).

It's the perfect rock to reveal the way toward lifting you into calming your mind, a more positive inner state, and assisting you to concentrate on what is important to you.

Quartz crystals can be used in these particular ways:

Employed in meditation crystal can allow your mind to soothe and unwind. The ideal structure and alignment of this crystal has the exceptional capability to deepen your meditation.

You can use a quartz crystal to save mental images your prayers, and feelings and enhance your working with your dreams.

A quartz crystal placed in front of your computer screen and will help defend you against electro smog.

How to Clean and the Crystal of Old Vibrations

Before use, it ought to be processed to remove any vibrations it has picked up for you in its way.

Those would interfere with the crystal with your optimistic exchange of electricity clear. You want the crystal to stay empty and clean to your functions.

You can make a cleansing ritual with the assistance of those four elements: earth, fire, atmosphere and water. I like the following procedure, which utilizes air:

1. You sit with your crystal in your hands and let your mind move silent, breathing in and out.

2. Hold your hand over the crystal and feel that the energy field.

3. Exhale and visualize blowing off the aged residual energy traces from the crystal.

How to Program a Crystal with Your Intention

Before usage, you will have made a mind picture of your intention, and target as described above.

It is advised to use a different crystal for every one of your objectives, so the crystal will fire up that specific vision each time you hold it.

The crystal ought to be programmed with goal or aim. Here is the way to do so:

1. Hold the crystal in both hands. Become aware of the crystal energy field between your two palms.

2. Focus intently on your intent, vision or goal. Imagine its clarity that is powerful, as though you are experiencing the goal has been accomplished. Feel the emotions of satisfaction and success.

3. Release your goal's picture using a breath out.

You have stored that idea those and form feelings in the crystal. This will fortify your field of anticipation, keeping you tuned into the world and calling the thing that you want toward you.

In programming your vision you have planted an anchor on your energy field that'll keep your subconscious mind tuned for your vision.

Ultimately, sit down holding your crystal clear, and imagine again when you achieve your objective, how great it will feel. Immerse yourself.

This is what I call "firing up" your eyesight occasionally. This permit it to flow and will raise your frequency.

Based on the Law of Attraction, if you want to permit the manifestation of your needs to flow for you, you want to be open, open minded, and about the ideal frequency.

Crystals are a highly effective mechanism for encouraging the process of reflection.

CHAPTER 7

THE BASICS OF CRYSTAL HEALING

Crystals healing can be linked back to the early Indians and Greeks who thought there were big gems that produces light to other world.

So using crystals for healing now isn't really all that fresh, however, it is still quite powerful and even more tasteful now.

We can find crystals around us every day and all the time, they are in computers, our watches, mobile phones and so forth.

Crystals, stones and stones are residing dense entities which give off energy and can balance areas of our bodies and air.

The application of stones or crystals within particular energy centers (chakras) brings light and color into the body's setting and also this light may encourage recovery.

Crystals are known to transform energy that stimulate healing. They can be used for recovery, and there is a transcendent character. Crystals are indicated to take care of a wide range of emotional and physical conditions including indigestion, insomnia, bursitis, headaches, forgetfulness, anxiety, depression, Parkinson's disease, hemorrhages, thrombosis, blindness, diabetes, rheumatism, and cancer.

All crystals possess diverse qualities and therefore are beautiful. It's possible to carry crystals inside pocket, set them in tub water, wear them on a string, or place them in your house to bring the energy of recovery in reach.

Different types and colors of Stones or crystals have been encouraged to possess different healing powers and some people today claim certain diamonds or diamonds transmit special energy that can be transferred to individuals to give protection against illness, restore health, and provide spiritual guidance.

There are a lot of applications that are great for crystals, you can set a crystal on your pets water bowl to keep water, fresh and valuable or you'll be able to place a crystal in your water bowl for purification and put crystals under cushions, on table tops place crystals around the home for stability hold one in your hand while stroking your cats or simply relaxing for psychic function, energy healing, and total wellness.

Once a month you need to place your crystals from sunlight to recharge them seeing as they may get so hot that they can begin a fire. Individuals who exercise various healing arts frequently for grounding themselves or the individual a bit shy.

Some healers like crystals with a great deal of personality and quirks in their appearance, also they enjoy them to become raw and unpolished.

When crystals are awakened it is said they have more female energy, known as yin so when the healer is focusing on healing feminine energy they'll use a crystal in the ground.

Energy and Protection

Everything inside the world is made up of energy and information. Energy vibrates at diverse frequencies but we couldn't observe this energy since they vibrate very fast. Due to the nature of our senses that are too slow to these vibrations, we can only receive chunks of information which permits us to be able to perceive the chair we're sitting, other people etc.

When you walk into it and an area feels like you can' cut the atmosphere with a knife', this can be referred to as negative electricity and likewise, if you go to a party, then you will feel excitement in the air - or even positive energy.

In precisely the same way, once we open up our energy facilities in meditation, healing, prayer, visualization or working with crystals, we're attracting energy vibrations to us (negative as well as positive). It's therefore necessary that we protect ourselves.

Grounding

Grounding is important to execute before you start to work with your crystals since it keeps you in contact with your surroundings.

Crystals will take you on a higher plane and if you complete your work, if you haven't grounded yourself ahead, you might encounter a drifting feeling and be psychological (like a recovery curve) as you've opened yourself up and could be vulnerable to other's negativity.

In other to ground yourself, you need to take three deep breaths, imagine that there are roots and sitting with your feet standing firmly on the ground.

They're growing down and down through the ground to the center of the ground to make certain you are really grounded. To ascertain your grounding, attempt to lift one of your foot. You know that you've grounded yourself correctly if you discover this difficult.

Prayer

Dear Universe I request that you surround me with the pure white light of your being that is divine.

Remove me from all vibrations to be dispersed in the world to anything else. Please put me in my very own bubble of protection that is complete.

Visualization

Visualize yourself standing at a Pink location, know that nothing could penetrate this bubble just divine light and love and bubble.

White is the color of heavenly protection and pink is your color of soul adore that is unconditional.

Blessing and cleansing of your Crystals

There are different ways in which crystals can be deciphered. But not every crystals can be set so it is important that you're careful about how that you wash them without being spoiled.

When crystals have been obtained and all cleanup has been completed. If your crystals were gotten elsewhere, then you'll have to get them cleansed.

With dust and pollution from the air, it's suggested that a baby's hairbrush is used to brush the crystals, which not just eliminates the dust but also stimulates the crystal.

Crystals also have to be blessed before use. The crystal has to be manually cleansed so that the crystal is ready to align with you.

A Blessing

Dear Universe,

I thank the mother earth for providing these crystals

for the benefit of humankind. I ask that the crystals be lucky to discharge all negative vibrations into the world to be spread without harm.

Working with Crystals

Before working with the crystals, follow the under listed basic steps:

1. Ground and Protect yourself

2. Bless and cleanse the crystals

3. Position yourself to the center by sitting with your eyes closed and seriously focus on your breathing for some moments.

When working with a crystal, gently hold the crystal with your right hand and start saying what you want to release all the negative vibrations without harm to any living thing.

Place the crystal Left hand and request the help that is specific you require. Work together with the crystal in every hand for ten minutes.

Crystal Healing Approaches

Explore Your Crystal

When you acquire a new Crystal you need to spend time exploring it. You'll discover that this develops your sensitivity.

Step 1 Look at your crystal from various angles, hold it in the hands noting and close your eyes.

Step 2 Hold the crystal in the two hands and breathe in the air penetrating inside the crystal and breath on the crystal so that you achieve different cycle of breath going inside the crystal building energy.

Step 3 With your eyes closed, Sit quietly and focus on the color you may imagine how the crystal feels in your hands And feel thoughts or any vibrations that cross the mind.

Step 4 Bend down and put the crystal in sense and your solar plexus how it feels, visualize the color of the form the crystal and any ideas that you pick up on.

Do this with your third eye, detect any changes.

Crystals, like Aladdin's lamp are greater than what they appear. Their aspects written by the Babylonians in parchment and have been carved in stone from ancient Egyptians.

Today the windows of Tiffany's and Cartier are a testament to our obsession with crystals and gemstones. The reason we trophy them has to do with how they make us feel we believe.

You will be told by any true scientist that crystals have charge or a power that is not too distinct from the body. So imagine what you can do with all this energy!

Studies indicate that when placed in water it changes the molecular structure or even the liquid, it emits vibrations and new technology can take photos of a crystals energy field.

So rather than using crystals transmit and to transduce energy in computers, TV's, and watches as they are used today- it is possible to use them attune to heal, calm and produce.

When the energy body or chakras of I or you, is upset or out of balance it's an immediate effect on our physical body- arthritis, muscle aches, acne - you name it!

A crystals individual properties may be used to

operate in harmony with the body to transmute or even amplify certain aspects in your energy body using 3 simple steps:

Crystals are not the same and it helps to be educated, when picking one. Like diamonds, clarity, color, cut and dimensions all make a difference.

But bear in mind that crystal has as much power only in various ways. Do a little reading and find what you're looking for. If you are feeling a little overwhelmed, don't forget the power of intuition!!

There are a number of ways to cleansing your crystal so that it is cleared of any previous vibrations or adverse charges and it is your choice to determine which one you feel is best.

My favorite method is to set the crystal in a bowl of water and leave it out during a waxing moon night.

Another way is to put it into a cluster of amethyst or clear quartz crystals for 12 hours. Remember your crystal is absorbing outside energy so it requires frequent cleansing for optimum use.

Your crystal can do a lot for you However; you have

to find out its strength and the reason why this stone that has been formed in the earth miles from your doorstep has come in your life.

Sure, you went out and purchased it- but it's a certain vibration and energy that is only one of a kind, just like you. Get to know its energy stream and your healing will do the job far better.

For:

Confidence: Carry or meditate with green jasper. This stone stimulates the heart chakra and the blood flow providing strength and courage.

Rejuvenation: Red garnet is a powerful energizing stone. Place a garnet at a glass of water for a moment and drink to give you a kick start to your day!

Relaxation: A method to achieve healing is when sleeping, by placing 8 amethyst crystals around you.

These crystals sleep and calm feelings and aid meditation. Try design patterns that are different.

CHAPTER 8
ADVANTAGES OF CRYSTAL HEALING

The Chi is the life force energy inside our own body. This Chi controls the different components of our presence and it had been said that crystals heal some pieces of our bodies.

According to belief, some crystals are concentrated on curing energies that were different. If you use the appropriate crystal on the chakra (which is the center of our body's power of energy), it will transfer an energy that heals and enhances your health and wellness.

Here are some unique crystals that may be used to cure components of our body.

* Beryl - can clean your throat And help improve your liver functions.

* Citrine- is a quartz that is yellowish That can help improve your blood circulation.

* Emerald- will help you get enough sleep and fight insomnia.

* Sapphire- will your clear Skin and enhance skin ailments

* Sodalite- reduces your blood flow pressure.

* Topaz- It assist the varicose veins.

The Advantages of Crystal Healing

When you purchase crystals for your own personal healthcare usage, don't forget to first wash them and wash well.

It eradicates any sort of negative energy that's been gotten from people who have managed this type of crystal. After washing the crystal, you need to plan it.

One method to plan the crystal Is to put in on your hands, hold it until you transfer your thinking to this crystal. This permits you to begin your healing powers.

This Idea of using crystals to medicate the body has been around for centuries. It is being practiced by a lot of people in certain states like India, and Egypt.

This idea may be strange to those who are not familiar with the 'chi' energy and unique practice. However, our body is made up of energy.

The crystals which we use to heal a specific disease, changes the power into an energy which penetrates the human body and resuscitates the systems.

Another way to program the crystal is to visualize an individual choosing the crystal up and seeing their miserable face transform to a joyful expression. Then visualize them having health that is exceptional and enjoying life.

The identical thing applies if you know someone who is suffering from any sort of illness. Consider these as a happy and healthy being. Picture them while you maintain the crystal rock.

These ideas are transformed into energy and whichever thoughts, whether negative or positive, it can be transferred to that person and stored in the crystal you are currently thinking about.

It is very important to believe in its own power, otherwise of shifting the energy, your effort won't work at all.

However, if you do think this, then it's possible to use the crystals more to heal mind, the body and well-being.

CHAPTER 9
CLEARING CRYSTALS FOR CRYSTAL HEALING

Crystal healing is a recovery technique where crystals are placed all around or on this receiver's body.

This healing technique has been since immemorial instances where it had been used to cure and to restore the body's energy.

These crystals assist the body to discharge and eliminate negative energy therefore promoting energy healing in the process.

Crystals have been described as character's gift to humankind to boost healing. They come in colors, all shapes, sizes and compositions.

Each and every crystal is unique in its own manner each crystal has an vibrational resonance.

Their mineral material, the colors they exude and

their geometry all contribute to the uniqueness of each and every one of those.

The human body has a vibrational energy system known as an intricate system.

As a result of nature, crystals are excellent electromagnetic conductors that are very much capable of interrelating with all the individual electromagnetic system.

Crystals are thought to carry vibration which will activate various energy facilities within the electromagnetic system.

Crystal Clearing

There are times when a crystal that attracted someone does not seem to do any longer. The crystal may have to be cleared when this occurs to be the situation.

It is important to have a rock or crystal cleared before using it because it is just then it may emit or release of its abilities.

When it is removed, a crystal that is will feel tingly

and cold, emits bright and positive emotions. However, a crystal or one that needs to be cleared may at times feel drained, hot or heavy.

There are ways crystals and gemstones are cleared and they comprise the following:

• Smudging - this is a quick way to clean a crystal or a gemstone where they're smudged with burning cedar or sage.

• Moonlight - that is also a method of clearing the crystals. It simply involves placing them out in the moon. Waning moons are recommended but any time can perform to dispel energies.

The timeframe will be dependent on the healer and sensitivity and also at the magnitude of stone or the crystal. Hanging a crystal on a tree out in the moonlight is a good idea.

Other ways include burying the crystal deep into the ground especially when clearing blowing off at the crystal with your breath and is required. It is believed that gemstones and the crystals will need to be cleared by a skilled healer

CHAPTER 10
CRYSTAL HEALING WITH QUARTZ CRYSTALS

A set of clear quartz crystals can be utilized to cure and to detox your emotional, mental, physical bodies, your Aura and the ethereal energy area. They may be used alone or along with minerals and other crystals.

These particular crystals enable the user to guide pure divine energy into and through their body.

Using crystals is a sure and effective way to improve the body's healing capability to process energy at a higher vibration rate.

Before you start using quartz healing crystals, it is advisable to allow the crystals to choose you.

Among the best strategies to differentiate which healing crystals are the ones for you. To be working together is to be given the frequency of the crystals.

If you are lucky enough to locate crystals in pairs, the majority of those "work" has been completed for you.

You just "ask" which pair of crystals resonate with you. Would you discern which ones are the ones for you personally?

Calm yourself, breathe exhaling slowly and move your left hand over every set. The crystals that radiate a warmth or distinct awareness of energy are those which resonate with you along with your own energy.

If you are unsure if what you are sensing or feeling is real, hold the crystals in the palms of the hands.

Bear in mind the point of this crystal in your left hand should be directed towards your wrist. The point of the crystal on your hand is to be directed towards your palms.

It's important for the quartz healing crystals to be held in each hand. When working with a pair of healing crystals, you turn into a channel to flow in to and out of your physical body. If the things are facing towards you or away it blocks the flow.

As soon as you have chosen which crystals you'll

work with. Cleanse before using them for the first 13, and re-charge the crystals.

To cleanse and re-charge your crystals, rinse them in warm water, then pass them or place them in sunlight light for a few hours.

Now you are ready to start using your healing crystals. Quiet your mind, hold your crystals breathe slowly and talk 3 times to the Invocation of Light.

You may talk it aloud or silently to yourself. The Invocation of Light is: I invoke the Spark in case Divinity inside, I'm a clear and perfect channel, Light is my guide.

You will begin to feel a soft tingling vibration. It may take a little practice for you feeling or to really feel the energy out of the crystals flowing though you.

Whether you sense or feel the crystals' energy flowing through you right away or not, trust it is happening.

The healing crystal in your left hand pulls in energy that is pure from the divine source. It takes all that is desired as the energy flows into, through and from your hand. Meaning, as you open yourself allowing Divine White Light to flow through you, all energy that has been accumulated, stored and become stagnant is purged from inside you and your Aura.

Remember your aura is a direct reflection of what is and is not happening in your physical body.

You can perform this simple technique on your own by standing up with your feet shoulder width apart, sitting in your mediation seat or placing down.

You may choose to let yourself at least 10 to 15 minutes the first few times. You will begin to notice how differently your system feels, as you become comfortable, gaining confidence in you.

Experience and you will start to feel peacefulness and harmony more often and for longer periods of time.

When you have finished your session, cleanse and re-charge the crystals. It's vital to boost your intake of water over the next 24 hours to finish your inner detox and healing procedure.

This simple crystal healing technique is quite effective. Your Everyday life will be enhanced by working with crystals and expand your Sense of conscious awareness.

CHAPTER 11
CRYSTAL HEALING AS AN ALTERNATE NATURAL THERAPY

Instead of healing method, or a technique for strengthening the human body, crystal healers have long been in existence for centuries.

Using patterns, the work with the aura of a body of a crystal healer, crystals helps it to heal in some way, whether physical or psychological.

Sometimes referred to as diamond treatment, the use of crystal healers is as widely diverse as the stones which are employed in this technique.

Crystal healers learn to heal a mind and body by enjoying with the crystals called chakras. A chakra is a term that identifies the spiritual energy that's present in everybody.

With seven main chakras through the body, each

chakra works together to form an individual's energy and if that's out of alignment it can bring poor or negative power to a individual either in mind or body.

The crystals the Energy and rather direct the flow of good energy back in the body which subsequently brings the balance the chakras naturally possess.

Ultimately, crystal healers utilize these stone to heal psychological discrepancies conditions, and misguidance that is religious.

History of Crystal Healers

Crystal healers have been discovered in virtually every culture throughout history from the Indian tribes to the people.

Although the actual originator of using crystals as bodily and mental therapy is unknown, it has been demonstrated that this technique has been practiced for centuries and is still used today all over the world.

Much the tomb of King Tut was surrounded by jade amulets that are thought to direct the soul after death.

The Chinese civilization greatly believe in using crystal healers, especially with the usage of jade and emerald which is considered to increase their memory and intelligence.

In different civilizations crystal healers would utilize all types of amulets, agate, lapis lazuli, amethyst and much more to assist with everything from stress to sickness.

The Benefits Crystal Healers Give to You

Crystal healers has a great number of benefits to assist ailments as well as the nature of a individual.

Some of the most effective benefits to crystal recovery are health as well as the usage of crystal therapy for personal development and vitality.

Healers work with you to promote change on your own and your brain and also to cure many bodily conditions when traditional medicine just doesn't seem to work or it has to be combined with holistic practices in order to spur on the recovery.

Other ways a crystal healer can benefit you is by alleviating stress, anxiety and depression, or just helping you to relax.

It can assist with menstrual problems, nausea, digestive issues, relief from pain, fatigue, memory loss, concentration as well as learning issues. It has shown great results with wealth building, connections and.

By working to cure the body, crystal therapy is a natural form of deep relaxation mixed with meditation that fosters the general immune system also makes the body work more efficiently. By balancing the mind it benefits the body.

It may boost creativity, enhance communication and even help with the development of your spirituality.

It's not advised that you replace medical therapy if it's needed, but it can give an increase to your health which can actually improve the body and mind. To anyone, or migraines offer you a world of benefits from raising feelings of love.

What Crystal Healers Can Do?

The act that a crystal healer performs is very straightforward. They set crystals on various areas of the human body, in a certain area of a room or anyplace that corresponds with the chakras that are out of equilibrium.

By assembling an energy grid of type to eliminate the terrible energy and bring in the good energy, crystal healers function to surround an individual with the healing energy they require.

This in turn removes the obstructed chakras from the air. The crystals give off healing vibrations for various treatments, by using the color of crystals which match up with all the color of the chakra. This brings about the positive vibrations that attract events from the life span.

Crystal healers work at a place in an area, usually of calmness that promotes comfort and quiet as well as calmness.

Fully dressed, the healer will inquire about that thing you believe is incorrect so that they can deduce exactly what crystals should be utilized and the chakras that needs to be unblocked as well.

Some of the most well-known gems doctors use is amber, selenite, increased lepidolite, and subilite although you will find many to pick from.

Each provides a curative property. By way of instance, amber helps with the energy that aids with love and self-esteem whereas the selenite assists the unblock energy of a person's greater awareness.

Crystal healers help an individual to heal themselves from within and it is a skill that everyone can learn.

In reality, there are lots of crystal healers' class workshops which encourage the total understanding of how crystal recovery can effectively alter a person's lifestyle and wellbeing.

Crystal healers workshops con help someone discover how to use visualization techniques as well as relaxation methods to help them eliminate the negative energy from their own bodies and balance the chakras to feel the positive energy transfer throughout the entire body.

CHAPTER 12
HEALING GEMSTONES AND CRYSTALS

The power of crystals and gemstones is a fascinating one, and remains to be completely explained. However, there is nothing to prevent you from trying crystals on your own, and experiencing their consequences firsthand.

Let us take a brief glance at what's involved in using crystals for healing and other life-improvement purposes.

The use of crystals is based on the concept of the body as an active system. Blockages can occur in the system, finally leading to physical disease or other issues.

Crystals have their own feature energies, which might be used to help dissolve blockages in the energy body, or to enhance its functioning.

Specifically, crystals tend to be utilized in

combination with the chakra system. Chakras are energy vortices which are observed in many places in the body, although most healers concentrate on the seven main primary chakras, which are located in a rough line between the crown of the head and the base of the backbone.

Chakra imbalances can lead to physical and psychological difficulties, and crystals may be used to assist 'song' the chakras and restore them to normal functioning.

How Is It Done

It's common to place crystals on the areas of the body during a healing session. In the event of using crystals for chakra work, they are normally placed in the area of the chakra(s) in question.

A healer might also use tools like a crystal wand to direct the energy in a more particular manner, or use a crystal pendulum to gain more information concerning the positioning of energy blockages or other issues.

Some folks also like to use crystal jewelry, or carry

small about with them, to benefit from the rock's properties through the day.

When using healing stones and crystals it is required to cleanse and recharge the stones. This can be accomplished by holding them under running water for a little, then placing them.

Which Stones Are Best?

Different gemstones have various properties, and stones that were so particular may be appropriate to certain functions.

Rose quartz for instance, has a very soothing, calming energy, which makes it great for dealing with emotional upsets, whereas carnelian is particularly prized for dealing with issues in the lower stomach such as reproductive or digestive problems.

Clear quartz on the other hand, is regarded as the 'universal healer', as this potent stone can be useful in a wide range of circumstances.

Many people have had good results which is why it

continues to be a remarkably common branch of complementary medicine.

Even though science is not as convinced with the attributes of the successes to the wishful thinking as it pertains to the individual.

Much like other 'option' pursuits where controversy exists, it's usually worth experimenting and making your own decisions, instead of taking the word of others as biases.

If you've got a physical or mental problem and are trusting that crystals might help, your very best plan of action is to visit a reputable crystal for advice, but to continue with whatever type of therapy your doctor has prescribed in the meantime

CHAPTER 13
CLEANSING CRYSTALS

To be able to remove any unwanted energy from a crystal, whether a crystal pendulum for divination purposes or a piece of crystal jewelry stones used for crystal healing, it's quite imperative that the crystal is properly vaccinated until it is used in any sort of healing or divination process.

Your crystals grapple with an energy frequency, which allows them to work in methods that are certain to heal, clear, and control people and environments.

The more they are used by you for healing sessions or round the house - the more vibrations which dull their ability are picked up by them.

It is like trying to use a paintbrush to paint a glowing new shade of crimson on a canvas after dipping it via black, green and blue. It just gets a bit brown in the long run.

So you have to wash that brush In between colors in

order to paint your masterpiece.

After some time, where your crystals are working hard you may begin to feel that they don't feel exactly the same once you hold them in your hand, or else they do not look exactly the same; maybe they lack the lustre they had initially.

You might even feel that they are effective during your recovery work. These are all signs that your crystal has to be cleaned. It's not hard, just a few basic rules to follow.

How often should I clean them?

This depends on how frequently you use them and how well they are kept. You will have a sense of when to do that. Get a feel of its energy in your hand when the vibration starts to wane, and you'll understand.

The best method is to get to some regular cleaning of the crystals. This way you won't neglect to do it particularly for those crystals that sit on a table in your sofa or sofa and are always on the job.

When should I wash them?

If you're currently cleaning them once, it's important you opt for the ideal time of day or the moon depending upon your method on cleanup Month.

Moonlight and dawn, the growing moon reflects new life and growth. Dusk or the waning moon represents a time of rest and removing of evil. Depending on the crystal's purpose you may choose one or the other.

Just how long do they need to be cleansed for? It is believed that whatever way of cleansing you opt to utilize, crystals need a 12-24 hour period to be completely clean.

It is almost always best to examine your crystal physically and psychically after every cleansing to decide if a longer time is required.

What different ways can I use to clean them?

There are many different ways to clean a crystal like moonlight, crystal clusters, pure and earth water sources. Earth and moonlight cleaning bathed in light for a particular length of time or buried in the earth.

Washing them rain water or in ocean or stream is another choice. However, whatever method you choose, it must always be blended with washing it in warm water and soap to eliminate the physical and the metaphysical dust and grime.

How do I recharge them are clean? Recharging crystals is not required, depending on the sort of crystal you are currently using. It's always nice to give your crystals a boost after cleaning them.

Combining another cleaning method with some time at a quartz or amethyst crystal cluster is my favorite choice however the crystals are being placed by another boost like a shot of espresso onto a drawing of this Reiki'Choku Rei' power emblem.

It's not hard to cleanse your crystals. It's definitely much harder work seeking to utilize that citrine you discovered under the mattress to capture the sun on your feng shiu room, or green aventurine covered in dust to cure your heart.

Now you understand the basics of cleansing your

crystals. Heal those precious gems well and they will do the same.

If curing stones are properly cared for, their abilities are extensive. Crystals help release energies, when applied therapeutically.

On the surface of the crystal, these energies that are unwanted accumulate in time and from the energy field that surrounds it.

It's like the mess on a desk may get in the way of your ability to work, the undesirable energies onto a crystal get in the way of its healing powers, and the stones must be cleansed.

If you use in crystal clusters your own residence or workplace to keep the atmosphere uplifted and clean of the room, cleanse the crystals each time you dust, or about once every couple weeks.

This will allow them to work in their finest. Healing crystals must be cleansed after every treatment session in which they are used by you. Three consequences might occur as indicated if you do not cleanse your crystals.

Negative energies the healing crystals pick up can be transmitted to the individual who receives the treatment. Second, these energies may be as the practitioner unconsciously picked up by you.

The crystal may continue to absorb the undesirable energies, which will further blur the crystal, making it less effective as a recovery tool.

The good news is that crystals respond to cleaning. Begin by cleansing your recovery crystals. It will easily remove the dust and grime that collects on the surface of the crystal. Use water from the sink only if tap water is non-chlorinated.

You will also need an old toothbrush and mild detergent or soap. Gently hold your crystal, place little detergent on the toothbrush, and then brush the crystal surface.

While the soap eliminates the physical dust and dirt from the crystals, the movement of the running water can help to remove unwanted energies your recovery crystals might have picked up during healing use, or while helping keep the energy in a room uplifted and transparent.

If your tap water has been treated, then pour into a big measuring pitcher. Clean the crystals together with the toothbrush before, but rather than using your faucet, rinse them by massaging the water that is purified.

Once the crystals are physically cleansed, you could clean their energy field employing a gem formula energy. This will remove energies the energy field could have picked up.

While using soap and running water above your crystals is successful for eliminating undesirable energies, this way isn't helpful in clearing the electromagnetic radiation that the crystals might have picked up from a patient's body and air in a treatment session.

Crystals also can absorb electromagnetic radiation from the immediate environments with relatively high electromagnetic fields.

A gem formulation EMR protection in spray form was made to handle this situation. Spray your crystals using this formula to rid them.

Next on your crystals using a gem formula diamond. This will clean accumulated energy in the crystals' patterns to bring forward advice about their true purpose.

You as the practitioner can decide the space from the crystals to hold at what, and the spray angle. The more carefully you personalize the spray cleanse, the more effective it will be.

By using soap and water to clean your crystals, and stone formulation sprays to clear them, your crystals will be able to share their maximum healing possible.

The Way to Tell Whether a Crystal Needs Charging?

Whenever you acquire a fresh crystal, it must be cleansed. All sorts of impressions will have been made on it between the time also the time that it came into your possession and it had been mined.

This energy is not necessary negative, although some of it might be. If there is no negative energy within your crystal, it's significant you alone and that it's tuned in to you.

Only then can the crystals are endowed by you together with your own energy.

A crystal will appear dull. This is quite obvious in crystal prisms, but could be seen in rocks like Jasper and Tiger's Eye. There are just two reasons for this dullness. One is that the crystal is. The second is the fact that it requires cleansing.

If you think your crystal requirements In a quiet location for 24 hours, leave it To break. If it's still dull after 24 hours, you can be certain it requires cleansing.

Even though nobody else has managed your crystal, it could have picked up other energies in the atmosphere around you, particularly if it's been used in intense or work. Those employed for crystal healing need cleaning frequently.

Bring or crystals used to shield energy to office or the house will likely have to be cleansed more often than the ones that brought out and just are kept in a place that is dark.

Again, check their glow --they need charging or

either tired if they're dull. Home or workplace crystals which are tired left and ought to be eliminate at a place to rest.

General Methods to Cleanse Your Crystals

How to cleanse and a crystal that is re-charge depends a lot on the sort of crystal. As each have their own attributes, they have their own requirements. But, there are general procedures which could be utilized.

Cleanse using a pendulum if you want to cleanse crystals at once, lay them into a ring. Hold a crystal probably rose quartz crystal over the stone or at the middle.

Move the pendulum over the crystals anti-clockwisely, for the amount of times that you think feels 'right'.

Gently dip the pendulum in chilled water the amount of times it was moved by you and shake to dry.

You can also move the crystal over the crystals but in a clockwise direction. They will be cleansed by the departure - the departure will enable them.

Cleansing with earth energies should you are close to place where ground energies are powerful, this is a great option.

Such places include fairy hills and stone circles, burial mounds. If fees are felt by it with positive energy, it's probably a good place.

Locate a flat rock and lay your crystals onto it. Lay the crystals in the base of a tall stone if a flat stone isn't available. Leave the crystals for 30 minutes while the earth cleanses and recharges them.

Cleansing with nature leave your crystals for 24 hours in moonlight, or in a rainstorm for about 5-10 minutes. The day of full moon would be the best time for cleaning crystals.

Utilizing amethyst wrap your crystals in a cloth along with a part of unpolished amethyst. Leave the crystals in a dark place for 24 hours to recharge.

Clean active' crystals at least after a week. It is best to have two that there's always one to use while one's being cleansed should you seek advice from your crystal daily.

The same goes for stones used in crystal healing.

It isn't hard and we owe it to our crystals. After all, they refuse to work for all of us.

CHAPTER 14
CLEAN AND CHARGE CRYSTALS WITH THE ABILITY OF EARTH, AIR, FIRE AND WATER

Crystals can enhance and empower every part of your daily life. Everything from relaxation methods to even discovering past lives or healing health issues!

When you discover a crystal or when a crystal finds you the very first thing you have to do is charge and cleanse your crystal clear.

There are several ways to do this. Listed below are a few options for you, listed with.

Natural water: flow, sea, waterfall, river. Hold crystal from the water and let it wash it over. Some crystals can become weak and damaged by water, such as talc.

Salt water: Equal parts chilled water and sea salt.

Some crystals cannot be placed directly in salt (like opals).

It may harm the crystal's structure, alter the end, or change the color of the crystal. You might set the crystal in a little bowl of water put that bowl into a bowl of salt so that the salt calms the crystal with no direct contact with the salt.

EARTH You can bury your crystal in plant or a garden and leave for 24 hrs. If you bury it in a garden, be sure to mark the place so you can find it again, and make sure any pets you have won't dig it up.

Crystal Cluster: Set your Crystal on a "chunk" or "bunch" of quartz or amethyst overnight. You might even use a glass jar of hematite stones. Also leave.

Rice: Set crystal at a small glass bowl with rice that is organic that is raw. The crystal from the rice for 24 hrs. When you're done, then discard the rice.

FIRE Candle flame: Gently old crystal and immediately hover it through the candle flame until they all burn out or surround the crystal with the light candles and leave it burning.

AIR Incense: (try lavender or sage). Hold the crystal and gently run it. Use a feather or hand to direct the smoke through and forward.

Smudging: Smudgestick and blow out, run the crystal over the smoke. Use your hand or a feather also. Sage is advised.

As soon as you have cleansed the crystal from all energies that you want to control your crystal.

To do this you simply hold the crystal in your hands while imaging all the negative energy exiting the crystal clear, see a dark mist float off or flake out, then fill out the crystal with glowing white light.

Watch the crystal filling And envision it radiating without a pure energy that is. Watch the crystal in your "mind's eye" as washed, clean and positively charged. Your crystal is a good idea to go and ready for use.

There are many ways to utilize crystals to empower and enhance your life. You can wear them, like in jewelry, and I am not referring to the expensive diamonds and rubies.

You may even make your own jewelry if you're the

type and are able to find beautiful crystals.

Crystals can be carried by you with you in a pocket or handbag for private security, put them around your house to lift negativity and maintain a joyful home.

You can fortune tell with them, meditate and even heal and diagnose your health problem. They can do amazing things and if you let them they could easily transform your life.

CHAPTER 15

USING CRYSTALS AS CURES AND ENHANCEMENTS

Feng Shui is a system of Improving the energy in your house to attract prosperity and decent fortune.

There are many distinct cures and enhancements you can make to reinforce the energy in your house and also my goal is to guide you through different kinds which are accessible to you.

In this chapter, I discuss with you a few very simple and effective improvements you may make using crystals that are generally used cures in Feng Shui.

Stimulating Chi

Possibly the Most common crystal cure would be to suspend a quartz crystal. This is a great cure if you want to excite the energy into your area or help it to flow naturally.

A common mistake that people make is to obtain a

large crystal, although size is significant it is not always true that bigger is better.

A crystal that is too big can overpower a distance and interrupt the power sending it zinging all around the area.

The optimum size for a crystal is one which is between 30mm and 40mm in diameter (roughly 1 inch to 1.5 inches).

Additionally with quartz that is clear because the clearer the crystal, the better, the best quality, most affordable crystal I have discovered is Swarovski which can be a little bit more expensive than some crystals but is well worth paying a bit extra for.

Energy Harmonization

If you believe that your home would benefit from energy harmonization then a great cure is to place a round clear crystal bowl in the center of your home within which you have put five crystals each of which represent one of the five components.

For wood usage a crystal this as green or jade fluorite. Fire is represented by purple or red crystals, fantastic examples here are Red Jasper, Red Jade and Amethyst. Earth crystals are brown or yellow crystals such as Citrine, Tiger Eye and Smoky Quartz.

For metal place hematite or moonstone and water is represented by both Jet and Lapis Lazuli. As this represents the movement of these elements the bowl in to which the crystals are put must be circular.

Attracting Love

If you want to attract love to your life, an excellent crystal cure would be to place two crystals. The top crystals to use here would be Rose Quartz or Amethyst.

Write down your hearts needs on a bit of paper, then wrap the paper around the crystals and place the crystals and paper at a red pouch, or cover with a red cloth.

Leave the crystals beneath your bed for 9 days before showing them prominently and taking out them.

Reduce your Internal Energy

To recharge your inner energy at the close of a long day, place a bowl of crystals from your bath. Fantastic crystals are Rose Quartz Jade, Moonstone and

Aquamarine.

Since you are relaxing with a long soak, have a crystal out of the bowl and hold it in your hands for a few minutes. You refreshed as you allow the power of the crystal flow through your body and will feel calmer.

Earning Money

To get a wealth treatment that is fantastic, place eight citrine crystals in a wooden box in which you have put a denomination note.

Set the box at the auspicious area of your house for wealth, this is the south east corner of your home or even the most auspicious place for wealth according to your kua number.

Once the box is put in place you must remember never to eliminate either the notice or the crystals.

CHAPTER 16
USING CRYSTALS WITH REIKI

The use of crystals is not essential for Reiki, however, many men and women are attracted to using crystals and revel in integrating crystals using their Reiki practices.

Here are some recommendations if you are attempting to decide which crystals to use in Reiki. You will want a different crystal for every chakra.

You can place the crystals on or near the body. For the crown, think about quartz crystal. For your brow, a dark blue or purple like amethyst would be suitable.

A blue green or light blue, like Aquamarine or blue lace agate, can be used for the throat area.

Like rose quartz on the heart area, attempt a pink crystal or tourmaline. The solar plexus area may benefit from a chartreuse or coral color.

Use peridot, malachite moonstone. A gold color works on the abdominal area. Try tiger's eye or amber.

At length, the pelvic space benefits from a shade that is profound so use garnet hematite, or obsidian.

Another way you can incorporate crystals into your Reiki practice is to set up a Crystal Grid. Opt for some crystals that you will use to make a pattern and you may then put this pattern beneath the Reiki table or seat.

The very first step after choosing your crystals would be to clean them. Hold them by one, after cleansing them and concentrate to flow through.

If you're a level one practitioner focus on directing your energy. If you are level two, you might use the symbols you have learned to channel the Reiki energy to the crystals.

Once you have channeled energy place them in a blueprint. A pattern to use is the Star of David design. In this design, place the crystals as the points of a Star of David with a single each for the foot and the mind and another four points as the buttocks and shoulders.

Feel free to experiment with Layouts before you find one which functions with you. Nothing with crystals is composed of rock.

If you channel Reiki for others, encourage them to bring their crystals or allow them to choose amongst yours.

Having something concrete to concentrate on the advanced equally in visualizing and focus as well as aids the beginner.

If you know what issues they are feeling, they can be guided by you to an appropriate crystal. By way of instance, suggest amethyst for someone who's currently suffering from anxiety.

Although crystals and Reiki are not traditionally used collectively, more and more folks are finding they complement one another.

If you are looking to expand your Reiki practice, incorporating crystals can be an enjoyable way to additional attune yourself to the universal energy.

Once you have learned the basic techniques of Reiki, see if they resonate with you and you are invited to find out more.

Crystals can be placed directly on a patient or within their setting. They may also be used near your computer to absorb power, around the home for purification, consume radiation and to absorb pollutants.

You can strategically place crystals for neutralizing geopathic stress and energies that are environmental.

Crystals could be worn as jewelry around your neck or carried in your pocket. You could submerge crystals on your bottles of drinking water purify and to strengthen it.

I employ crystals in all not all my healing sessions. If I feel that you would be skeptical about crystals, I am much less likely to utilize them.

On the flip side, many patients are extremely keen on finding more about crystals, therefore that I use them liberally.

In the ground chakra located beneath the feet, place a grounding stone like smoky or hematite quartz.

I generally do this during every recovery because these stones are helpful for collecting any unwanted energy swept in the patient's air during recovery. It is especially important to cleanse these stones following every healing, as they function as a receptacle for damaging or unwanted energy.

Crystals can be efficiently used on each of the chakras. I've included just a few to give you a flavor of diversity and the variety of recovery stones available to us here on earth. For root chakra, a smoky quartz can assists in purifying and grounding.

You can also choose a crystal such as carnelian which is. Red jasper grounds energy and may also be utilized for healing the circulatory, digestive and sexual organs.

If your individual has specific issues, choose crystals for their specific healing attributes. Let me let you cleanse your healing crystals after every use. Run them under new water or wash them.

You can hold them on your hand purify and to energize. With Reiki 2, imagine Sei He Ki symbols and the Cho Ku Rei penetrating and enabling every stone. You can put your crystals in the sunshine to assemble the sun's energy and purify them.

For sacral chakra, you can choose red Jasper for improving relationships and curing of body sexual organs. Orange calcite removes fear, helps overcome depression, balances the emotions and for healing the reproductive system, gallbladder and intestinal disorders like irritable bowel syndrome.

Yellow tourmaline arouses the solar plexus and is helpful to enhance power. It also heals liver, the stomach, spleen, kidneys and stomach.

Another gorgeous rock is that the tiger's eye that works on overcoming self-criticism, manifesting the will and strengthening self-worth. Crystals of a gold or yellow color are suitable for positioning on the solar plexus chakra.

When scanning the body of the patient at the start of a recovery, you will find weakness or a blockage. In such case, place the crystal on the chakra during the healing.

The crystal functions as the "third hand" during the duration of the recovery process. When doing this, many people report that they believe my hands on one of their chakras once I've moved to a recovery position that is different.

I normally place quartz rose on the heart. The stone which I love most was a rose quartz and I usually carry it with me all of the time. It was used by me for every healing. Finally I decided to give it to a friend.

It was the finest present I had in sharing and my possession it with a friend was the main thing that I could do with it.

Rose quartz also symbolizes purifying the heart at all levels such as love of self and unconditional love. You will attract loving relationships, as you reinforce your love of self.

Rhodonite is another pink rock that may be placed directly on the heart chakra, or just over it.

Emotional wounds heal, ease forgiveness and transmutes emotions that are painful. Green stones such as moss agate walnut and tourmaline may also be used effectively when working within the heart.

It would be very embarrassing if you do not place a crystal right. It's better to put your crystals or to one side. I normally use a quartz that I got in Argentina in the mysterious town of Capilla del Monte.

It is used by me specifically issues. For a time, this was my favorite stone, therefore that I always carried it in my pocket.

As I got used to it, I felt confident using it in every healings. This demonstrates that confidence I have in the healing energy capability of a crystal, and affiliation with it, enables your own crystals and you to be effective at curing.

Naturally, amethysts do have a high spiritual vibration. It strengthens intuition, common sense, spiritual insight, and psychic ability. It is always acceptable for use with the brow chakra.

Purple amethyst is useful as it connects the emotional, mental and physical bodies with the spiritual, the crown chakra.

It cleanses the air and transmutes negative energy. It's one of the most spiritual stones. I would suggest amethyst if I had to recommend one stone for meditation practice and the recovery.

If you decide to purchase stones for your own use, take a look at a gem shop and examine their inventory.

Pick any rock up that you find appealing and hold it in your hand. It may be your stone, if it resonates with you.

Talk about the qualities of the stone with the retailer or study more about esoteric attributes and its therapeutic.

Employing a combination of touch, wisdom and intuition, you are going to discover that the crystals suitable for you.

You use it to read which crystals will be most in tune with your personal energy and can bring your pendulum to the gem shop with you.

On a note, be aware of the shapes. Highly polished stones which produce beautiful bracelets, but to me, all that processing and polishing divert from the pure, natural aesthetics of this rock will be found by you.

Thus, I prefer a demanding, unpolished stone as it was found from the earth. On the flip side, crystals can be artistically crafted to spheres wands or hearts. My experience is that crystals shaped into balls could be a bit problematic.

No sooner did they choose a deep breath when crystal went rolling off the chest proceeded to roll away across the room.

CHAPTER 17
ISOCHRONIC CRYSTAL ACTIVATION FOR CLEANSING AND CHARGING CRYSTALS

Isochronic crystal activation might seem enthusiasts that are even to other healing that are new but it has been gaining ground because it was made available.

We've known crystals besides being decorations and accessories to be used for their therapeutic purposes. They serve an even better purpose than to be gratifying to your eyes.

Crystals are the gifts and of nature thereby will come with vibrations and many energies.

Cleansing and purging of those crystals are required beforehand in order to get the maximum out of them and after which, you can really program or tune your crystals to serve certain functions to influence and develop some area of your life.

Trusted and there are old methods as it continues to supply methods of doing things, introduces us.

Tones are utilized to clean and trigger gemstones and crystals. Just as you listen to specific isochronic tones to bring about favorable changes on your wellbeing so that the crystals imbibe certain frequencies and supply you with efficient healing crystals and gemstones.

You can add crystals to self-development practices and your recovery processes readily.

Cleansing and charging crystals

You will have the ability to locate loads of information about how best to cleanse and moisturize your crystals.

A few agents used to perform this are sea salt, moonlight, sunlight, water and even dried herbs.

For sure they have worked since individuals continue to use them now but insignificant and random energies and frequencies contribute to inconsistent outcomes.

Isochronic crystal activation gives you control over the frequencies and pruning to a direction of your crystals and gemstones.

It's within your power to emphasize what energies can operate with the properties of gemstones and your crystals.

This Procedure allows you to harness the power of the crystals. You are able to fortify them via charging with the assistance of isochronic tones, once you know the qualities of the crystals of your choice.

Crystals sets

If you do not know anything, it's possible to simply buy crystal sets which come with a cleansing and activation CD and directions.

If you read a bit about crystals ahead since their properties will enable you to know easily which one you would love to work with it would help. Make sure that you do your research and do not take anything.

CHAPTER 18
CRYSTAL PENDANTS AND THEIR EFFECTIVENESS

Crystals possess the ability to change and influence lives. If you ever see somebody putting on a crystal necklace then do not think it is solely meant for fashion.

Most people so much believe in the worthiness of crystals and the miracles that they performs.

If you're totally ignorant about the crystals' worthiness then keep reading this chapter to figure out the forms of crystals using their meanings.

The Heart Shaped Pendants

As all heart contours do the contour will attract the energies. Assist can be also found by those with negative emotions.

This assists one to recuperate from his or her state of distress and despair, melancholy, pain and has a healing effect on the wellbeing. This crystal pendant is also thought to be for raising a person's fertility great.

The Cube Pendants

This shape results in a significant kind of energy. They have a stabilizing effect on the people together. If they are programmed in that order, these crystals help achieve certain intentions.

The Pencil Pendants

Like the pencils, they are long, slim and normally have a pointed end. The end is dull. The energy employees use the crystal pendant to make. They can be used for ordinary use by the crystal healers.

The Egg Pendants

This crystal pendant caters to the aesthetic attractiveness of a person. Also the ones who practice acupressure as well as the reflexlogists use such crystals.

The egg shaped energy help rectify that over time and also may find out an imbalance in your system.

The Pendulum Pendant

They can be made to wear a necklace. Additionally they can be used as a pendulum. If you're wearing them then they can be a healer and protector for you.

This crystal necklace also identifies any imbalances which you're having in your physique. The hypnotists and the healers utilize the flux crystals for many purposes.

The Wand Pendants

The crystals have a round end along with a pointed end. The rounder facet is wider. They are made artificially. They're great because they can guide the energy flow in a specific direction.

The Laser Wand Pendants

They've a clear color. The duration of the crystal pendant is extended with a thin tip. The energy concentrates on the strategies and this type of crystal is quite much helpful.

The power healers use them mainly. If you're utilizing them afterward do have direct and positive intentions.

If you are looking from any of these bracelets you can purchase them on line. There are lots of internet crystal pendant websites that sell very good quality pendants of crystal.

CHAPTER 19

THE USE OF CRYSTALS AND GEMSTONES AROUND THE HOME

Few men and women are conscious of the fact the very crystals that they have selected to decorate their home with due to their attractiveness in fact are contributing to the overall atmosphere of the environment.

For each crystal has its own properties that are distinct; and each color will contribute to those properties too; changing the air from subtle yet noticeable ways.

When an individual wishes to purchase crystals, it is a good idea for them to do a small research not just on the sort of crystals they need to buy, but the colors as well.

For example, if someone puts violet crystals and gemstones throughout their residence will become more perceptive than they had been previously.

Gemstones and yellow crystals are known to promote digestive aid; so they need to be placed in the kitchen or dining room to make sure that individuals avoid digestive upset while they are currently eating.

The soft, pale pink crystals and diamonds like rose quartz ought to be utilized in a kid's bedroom, for they are calming.

When someone wants to buy crystals to use in jewelry, particularly when they desire to use rose quartz in something such as a necklace or ring, they should first make sure the gem they're interested in appeals to them. For styles and cuts of crystals and gemstones are offered for use in jewelry.

That is because different shapes and styles offer different aesthetic appeal. Rose quartz in particular is offered in rather a huge variety of styles and acts as a beautiful stone to exhibit in crystal jewelry, whether as the attention rock or simply as an accent to a beautiful ring, pendant or broach.

Crystal jewelry is something can be worn by people

of all ages, particularly if the crystal in question is increased quartz.

This is an incredibly versatile stone which can be used in any kind of jewelry; ranging from a pair of earrings or a dainty ring to the large center stone for a stunning and beautiful necklace.

Rose quartz crystals comes in many colors and shapes; making it among the most appealing stones of times.

Individuals who spend time before they opt to buy crystals researching their purchases find themselves intrigued by the information that is offered to them.

For not only can they discover special properties they may not have been aware of; but they'll also find interesting properties regarding their favorite color too.

1 example of this is: if somebody prefers the color grey above all others, they will find they like a complicated shade that also encompasses puzzle and sorrow.

Crystals and colors play with a very role in everybody's' everyday lives, even if they don't immediately realize the subtle changes which take place. It is a smart choice to become informed concerning the crystals in question.

You may find it hard to think, but minerals do and crystals have healing properties. Although the science isn't well understood, there are lots of individuals, cultures, and history which advocate the usage of gems and crystals for particular uses. Let me explain the fundamentals.

Have you ever slept with a crystal under your pillow? Try it with amethyst or malachite and you'll notice a clear effect.

Open up those crystals will help cure your psychological, physical, psychological, state. Once you do, you will have a new method for and a new hope through crystal healing.

Americans these days simply think in science. Some of it has been proven, although well, that which IS science. Take our ideas for an example. We can't read them or show them, although we have ideas.

Here we receive the "gray Place" of metaphysics. To

believe in Crystals that Heal, you must know that Metaphysics is science. We don't have enough equipment to measure the greater activities of vitamins and minerals. Plus, we are not looking for this.

How do crystals heal, then?

Science has shown that all things are energy and energy vibrates. Science has also proven that ideas, prayers, and other things that were surprising can change those energy vibrations.

Crystals hold a vibrational pattern that affects the vibrations and frequency of water in addition to those of individuals (and their bio-electro-magnetic field.

Various crystals and minerals basically holds a distinct vibrational patterns, so by making use of different gemstones, you can affect different parts of the mental, physical, emotional, and spiritual anatomy.

The longer you're exposed to a specific kind of crystal, the more it may have an impact on you, as your patterns align with the crystal's vibrational patterns.

Recognizing that the vibrations of minerals and gemstones are about as fine as those of ideas and emotions, is easy to see why believing in the healing power of crystals would increase their effectiveness.

And thus does holding or wearing a crystal up against the skin or ingesting a Gemstone Elixir,

The duration of time a person is in contact with a crystal is a factor in how much affect the crystal is going to have.

Crystals have different healing abilities. They are believed to have therapeutic effects when crystals are placed in points where the energy is carried out, known as chakras. They rejuvenate the system and permit the individual to achieve well-being and better health.

Crystal healing has three actions that are important. The first one is the cleanup process. The crystals during this process would try to remove the energy blockages which could be the reason for the illness.

The crystal has to be in touch with the person who is getting the recovery process in this time.

The healing crystals will need to be placed in direct

sunlight every week. This in precisely the same recharge the energy of the crystal and could cleanse.

The second step would be the harmonizing and integrating process. The changes are contained on your being. There could be some adjustments on the person's part. Why? Since the toxins are being flushed out of the body.

Stability is the next step. In this measure, the modifications are accepted by the body and becomes stable due to this change.

Body would mean that your body is able to endure pressure and the harsh surroundings even.

But the stabilized stage will wear off and you would want to put in your recovery crystals to get back on your feet.

Crystals that are different can cure various kinds of illnesses. Here are some crystals and the advantages they can give into the body.

• Amethysts are rocks assist in anger control and even that are generally utilized to tackle problems with blood sugar, nightmares.

• Blue green aquamarine stones are ideal for reducing anxiety, boosting immune system and the immune.

• Coral stones would increase your metabolism procedure

• Diamonds would help in construction your confidence, confidence and clarity.

• Emeralds do help in managing depression and also improve eyesight.

• Sapphires can as well helps to reduce inflammation.

• Jade do treat illnesses and impotency. It can help to talks about leadership and love and at the same time never afraid in the menstruation for women.

• Rubies are also for clearing or cleansing the blood.

• Quartz Crystal Enables a man to be able achieve peace, to heal inside and forgive and be kind.

Crystals naturally have healing skills, but not be complacent and try to cure your sickness. Obviously, you will require medical care.

Crystals could help increase the strength of the body

and solve some issues; it has a natural energy which could help us be rejuvenated. Crystal jewelry are not for accessorizing anymore, the only, it's gone deeper than that.

CHAPTER 20
ADDING CRYSTALS & STONES TO YOUR MEDITATION EXERCISE

I've always loved crystals. I like to be surrounded by them, place them through meditation on Chakra points and I really like to hold them in my hands, and I love to wear them.

When I first learnt working with crystals, I found myself drawn to amethyst quartz and I think that is because those crystals pack a punch that was vibrational when it comes to opening up the 6th and 7th Chakras, that helps you open up to Spirit.

I am certain that working with amethyst and quartz helps me become a clearer station today as I continue to "take dictation"

It didn't take long to understand that holding and/or wearing crystals greatly enhanced my meditation and I think I understand why:

(1) The energy of these crystals merges with our field, helping to maximize our general degree.

(2) The color vibrations of the crystals raise healing energies and the force round the body.

It has been a great experience that meditating with crystals has helped me to attain a balance of energy - I feel after working and working with stones and my crystals.

This is because we can choose certain crystals to achieve specific goals-it just requires a bit of research on reading or line books to learn the attributes of each stone.

I discovered it very simple to incorporate stones and crystals into my daily meditation practice, and below are some tips for those of you that want to give it a try:

Opt for the crystals you want to work together;

Hold on the crystals, wear them, or place them around you at which you are able to view them;

Meditate as usual.

I have to be habitual, because I've used essentially the

same crystal meditation for many decades! I began this practice to allow me to wake up higher consciousness centers and helps attain a state of consciousness.

If you want to try it, you only want one crystal-a clear quartz point maybe not a round flat rock, and also you get to lie down-which is quite relaxing after a tough day on the job

Lie face up;

Set the point of this clear quartz at the very top of your head;

Meditate as normal (try to work up to at least 15 - 20 minutes).

It's an incredibly power meditation, and to help ground the experience and draw it into physical reality (which makes it easier to recall your experience so you can set it in your meditation journal), try adding two crystals into your meditation:

Put an amethyst crystal on your eyebrow (Third Eye) and the citrine crystal onto your own navel (Solar Plexus).

The amethyst and citrine should be mild and on the flatter side so they do not distract you or roll during meditation. Meditate for 15-20 minutes (or longer if you've got time.

About that meditation journal - Through time, I've kept a meditation journal in which I record what and how I felt as I labored with various crystals and stones-I highly suggest since it will allow you to recall which crystals work best for different purposes keeping one.

To help get you started, here's a bit from my workshop notes and personal experiences concerning the 3 crystals used in the meditation summarized previously:

Quartz

Radiates the Divine white light and allows the consumer to work with that mild. It is generator, amplifier, conductor and a receiver of energy.

It greatly help in opening psychic centers, thereby assisting one to meditate. It's really helpful when utilized through meditation and when working with one or Spirit's higher self.

Amethyst

Among the stones that are finest for meditation and it works especially well when put over the third eye (between your eyebrows).

It is a stone--it works in planes, and the Spiritual to present balance, calm, patience, and peace.

Emotionally, amethyst can help heal grief and losses. Amethyst promotes peacefulness, happiness, and contentment. It brings internal strength and psychological stability.

Citrine

Citrine is great for dissipating negative energy, and may be utilized to clear negative energies in the human body and the surroundings.

It enhances mental clarity, confidence and nourishment while helping to relieve anger, self-doubt, and depression.

Citrine is and is a stone that is joyful also thought to promote success, prosperity, and prosperity!

To locate stones and the crystals that are right for

you, hold them in your hands with your fist closed.

You are going to sense a vibration in your hand when it's the best one for you. Consider adding them to your own meditation and feel the difference,

CHAPTER 21
SELECTING YOUR FAVORITE CRYSTAL

The power of crystals and their beneficial health aspects are understood for centuries.

The early Egyptians and Greeks, utilized crystals broadly as equally charms and amulets. Native Americans and Chinese, used them extensively.

Everyone should have a number of crystals they were at least touch each and every day, here I am going to explain a little bit about how to choose a crystal that's best for you.

The most important factor to remember when selecting a crystal is to follow your instinct. Do not take other peoples preferred and expect it to be your own favorite. It does not mean it is ideal for you although they may like it's appearance or feel.

You will know when a crystal is right for you, the closest thing to this is 'love at first sight' you'll feel an immediate attraction and sense of health when you hold it. Selecting your crystals ought to be a joyous experience, if you are unhappy with a particular crystal then it is not right for you.

And remember that is perfect for you may not be ideal for you. Your energies will change over the duration of your own life and you will have to modify and replace your crystals as you change and grow. That is another component of the fantastic journey.

There are four procedures that are basic to choosing a crystal, they might not all work for you, so if the first one fails proceed on to the last, and do not forget to trust your intuition - it won't fail you in the event that you believe in it.

1 - Sit on the ground with a collection of crystals. Close your eyes, take a couple of deep breaths and relax. Open your eyes and pick up the very first crystal your eyes are attracted to. This is the visual way of choosing a crystal.

2 - Follow the directions, nevertheless don't open your eyes relax and with your eyes closed run your hand

very slowly over the circles, without bothering them. Focus on the energy emanating from the crystals and when you are feeling one that is in tune with your energy and vibrations pick this up.

3 - With the crystals on the floor around you, shake your hands aggressively to get rid of any vibrations and take a couple of deep breaths. Then pick every crystal up and sense its own psychic vibrations. With you will be your crystal, the one that you feel is moving in resonance.

4 - This process requires a partner that will assist you. Put your arm out flat with your shoulder and ask your spouse to put two hands on your upper arm and then gently push your arm down. Pick a crystal up clear and hold it.

Concentrate on its energies and consult your partner to push down your arm, repeat this with all crystals. It feels strong and if your spouse can't transfer your arm you have found the crystal for you.

Crystals can improve your quality of life, when you find your crystal, be sure to use it to its entire potential, and after you are feeling a loss of appeal to a particular crystal, pass it on to a friend and find another.

CHAPTER 22
EXPLORING CRYSTALS AND INTUITIVELY

Your goal might be to research the crystals you own and find their electricity and possibilities.

You may have something in particular you want help with, such as curing a spiritual, emotional, psychological or physical dilemma or ailment.

Your goal might be to increase psychic abilities and your intuition, connect to your higher self and guides, and essentially discover your spiritual self. No matter what your goal is, the way to approach your crystals is simple!

1) You make a decision to strategy your crystals to select one to work with, no matter what your objective is.

2) You Opt for any crystal that appeals to you right at that moment, without doubting or looking up

information.

3) You maintain that crystal to get a moment and decide how you want to utilize it.

Maybe you'd already set this purpose in step one for example if you're picking a crystal to take in the bath with you or wanting a crystal to meditate with.

Whatever method and crystal you use, be aware that you're indeed getting some advantage from this particular crystal.

If you follow your gut feeling about what you're doing and just let it flow, too following your gut feeling about when to put the crystal etc., you will never go wrong and it is this easy - reach out and listen.

When you decide to use your crystals in any way, your energy reaches out, with or with a particular intention, and you'll select.

Remember there are many ways crystals can help us by increasing or quieting our energy, providing security or grounding, restoring balance/healing, etc.

Some will create a sense of motivation or inspiration;

a few will help you feel safe, less fearful and more confident; a few will attract your attention to emotions or pain that you need to heal; a few can reinforce positive feelings that will help you deal and get your life going in the ideal direction.

Whatever way someone can be away Unbalanced and track crystals might help restore the strain and attention.

Whatever aspect of your life and yourself you wish to improve, crystals might help encourage this procedure and fortify kickstart.

No matter what goal you have, simply opt allow yourself to be drawn to them and to choose one or more crystals.

Seeing or feeling the advantages

Some people will feel or sense the crystal affecting them in some way when they are used by them.

This will usually be most powerful at times when you are deeply relaxed and are more responsive, e.g. in meditation, while sleeping and through fantasies, when relaxing while stones are placed in or around you.

At a later date when they recognize the changes which have taken place within themselves, the ramifications may only be accomplished for many.

This could be a change of prognosis or attitude, a sense of being lighter and more focused more at the present than previously, more positivity and motivation in life and above all, feeling happy within yourself and attached to the bigger picture so you move more unconsciously through life and with greater link to your true self. Is not this the whole goal anyway?

When we connect within to discover who we are, all else in life falls right into place. If you feel light years away from such self-discovery at this point in time, ask your crystals assist you with this, but you need to also make the time to attain some stillness in your life or you will continue being preoccupied and busy, continuing to avoid yourself.

Stillness is Vital

Begin by using it to sit still with a crystal and explore it. Gaze at it, pay attention to your breathing, and allow yourself become one with that crystal and just let your thoughts float away. Using the crystal as a focal point enables your mind to achieve your eyes a little easier than if you simply shut and have a variety of images and thoughts crop up.

Concentrate on that crystal, see its everything blurs and let go fuzzy. Allow it to be. If thoughts do not get frustrated with yourself, just return your focus to your breathing and the crystal and keep.

Doing this for even 5 minutes a day, together with whatever crystal you decide on, can help your personal and spiritual journey in immense ways.

As we are creatures of this 'active mind', it is one of the things that are most difficult to calm that mind, but when we do we've a whole world of possibilities open up to us things which bring us great realizations and joy.

You'll never look at yourself or the world the same. But that's for you to discover and that I wish you well with it!

Rather than looking at a crystal like amethyst and saying "this crystal has XYZ properties", I believe it's a lot more useful to check at groupings of crystals which will give you an notion of the general qualities of the crystals based on their colors.

Colors - generally these have a higher or faster vibration since the lighter the color, the quicker its energy vibrating or is currently resonating.

The vibration of light at different frequencies is exactly what allows our eyes to see colors that are different in the first location.

Light colored crystals are fantastic for meditation, psychic and spiritual exploration and cleansing energy and advancement in addition to clearing.

Examples are pale blue white, clear and green, as well as crystals. Important keywords for light crystals include: awareness, ether/spirit/air (including thoughts and feelings), clearing/purifying.

Dark colours - Coloured crystals are fantastic for grounding, healing the body, coping with material issues, feeling secure and reducing anxiety.

Examples are earthy colors such as red, brown, orange and yellow, plus other colors such as black, gold and silver. Major keywords for dark crystals include:

recovery, protection, grounding, vitality.

Nature connection - Even though all crystals have the earth and nature, a few crystals have more of a nature sense, whether it's to do with their earthier colors or their patterns. Examples of nature crystals are ocean agate, tree agate, various agates like moss agate and so forth.

Unakite is a combination of Pinky-orange and green that always makes me think of character and the heart (because of the colours), so my sense is that unakite aids with a feeling of connection to all nature via the heart, fostering a sense of oneness which you can link with well by using unakite in meditation, but you may also realize that carrying it with you throughout the day helps you've got insights to the connectedness of life and the small things you experience throughout your day.

You can be guided by the appearance of the crystal to understanding possible applications and functions. The Significant key words for nature crystals would be: oneness, link, compassion

Keep it flexible

The groupings are generalized rather than restrictive, so don't hesitate to use any crystals because you are drawn to. I am a big fan of exploration and getting enjoyment. See what happens when you put a crystal at your third eye such as.

You're not restricted from the chakras in using crystals that are coloured with the coloured chakras or energy centres.

You might find that you putting a dark crystal in your brow helps your mind become concentrated and gives you a feeling of groundedness and are feeling light-headed. By placing the crystal in feet or your root chakra you do have to floor your energy.

CHAPTER 23
ATTRACTION'S ROLE IN SELECTING YOUR CRYSTALS

Have you ever thought about why you are attracted or attracted to stone or a crystal and not to another?

Maybe this particular crystal trying to get your attention as it has lots is calling outside and recovery.

Actually this is a good indicator of the crystal for you at this moment. More often than not you feel a magnetic pull or sense a strong urge to touch or pick up a crystal when you see it.

Being attracted to certain crystal or stone is not all that different to those occasions when you've been drawn with whom you have then formed a friendship and connection.

Often it's their bodily appearance that catches your attention; nevertheless remember that a crystal may not be attractive; pretty and all shiny, indeed it might look regular and plain.

It is power and healing properties which induce it to be chosen by one rather than your attraction to its external appearance, or the crystals energy shaking.

Each crystal has its own innate personality and character traits that are underlying and as all of us know we get along with and work with specific personalities than we do with others.

The more you learn about crystals and open yourself to their vibrational healing energies that the further you will be drawn to crystals. As time goes on you may learn how to trust this.

You could say that this leaves us with a question - do they pick you, or Do you pick your crystals? Or is it perhaps a two way road?

Discovering what this crystal may need to offer.

Now that this relationship has begun, you can confirm this by sense its energy clear and simply holding the crystal.

Sensitivity to vibrations or energy varies from person

to person. However, all you have to really know is that when a rock feels right when you manage that, then there's more to it than simply - attraction at first sight. It appears it's not right for you and you're not in sync if it doesn't feel right, leave it .

Further, discovering exactly what this stone has to offer and what its ability or purpose is can be accomplished commencing with it to bond and by holding it.

Gifting a Crystal.

Occasionally a particular crystal lets you know that it's not for you but for somebody else, then opens a dialog to speak or gets your focus. Or from the start you know.

Force that is universal or nature has a way of delivering the stone support and to heal you, or in this situation needed by somebody that you know.

For example, while picking up and handling image or your buddy's name will enter your thoughts and you also intuitively know who it is intended for. You have been recruited to provide this stones healing energies.

Follow through if you are in a place to do it and make a present of it. Tell your buddy that the rock made you believe of them and you'd like them to possess it. It is the fact after all.

If you're intentionally picking a crystal just hold their image and name and allow the magic of fascination to develop into play. For them will be, you will come across the stone that is most appropriate.

CHAPTER 24
GENERAL CRYSTAL MAINTENANCE OF YOUR FINE CRYSTAL

Glass with a lead oxide that is particular is called crystal. By integrating lead oxide to the glass results in a much greater vibrancy, improving density and superior representing features. Fundamentally, greater colour refraction means there's more lead from the crystal.

Not crystal is created both, though. Some crystal is heavier, creating more fat, since it's made out of a larger percentage of lead.

A crystal piece blown by hand will have some air bubbles. These tiny air pockets will be the effect of the accumulation of very small air bubbles generated during creation of this crystal.

The sole way these minuscule Pockets of air can be detected is to hold the piece up to a powerful light source. It is actually 1 manner.

Hand-craftsmanship can be identified by particular markings called flow lines and chill marks. All these are by no means considered imperfections, and are merely methods of determining the authenticity of a piece that is handmade.

Flow lines, miniature air pockets, chill marks, and other insignificant variations will always be current, even in the most lavish crystal. It's unavoidable when the piece was handmade.

Although heavier on account of crystal, the lead is milder. Dust can harm your crystal, so knowing the proper cleaning and care of your crystal is essential to prevent chipping, abrasions, fractures, and scratches.

This is some overall crystal maintenance.

Place crystal glassware.

Glasses should always be stored bottom-side down, which can support the weight of the glass much superior than the rim.

Don't move crystal from cabinet to table in a single

big "armload." Each glass separately.

Broken crystal may be salvageable. Designed epoxy may be used to re-bond a crystal piece. Set the bit in sunlight to help the holding power of this while.

Here are some cleaning techniques for crystal.

Dust can render abrasions and noticeable lines on your crystal. Clean gently with a lint-free drying cloth, using soap.

Do NOT use ammonia glasses which have patterns or rims etched in golden. Keep to the soap that is gentle.

Glass produced with direct oxide is called crystal. Putting lead oxide into it, which results in a brightness and color fraction creates denser glass.

Basically, more spectacular prisms of color are achieved by increasing the oxidation. Not all pieces of crystal are completely alike. Weight is carried by some crystals, because of the extra lead.

A glass handmade in crystal will almost always have some very small air "holes". As air is shaped these little air bubbles are caught inside the glass and carry of sculpting the crystal piece by the heating process.

The way that these slight variations in the crystal can be discovered is by placing it under lamp. Crystal specialists use this method to see as it may be labeled, whether an item was actually handmade.

Being made by hand can be determined about the outer surface of the crystal by particular tell-tale signals termed stream lines and cool marks.

Having any of those markings doesn't indicate the crystal is defective or inferior it's simply another way of authenticating work.

Chill marks, flow lines, nearly air bubbles, and other trivial things will found one of the priciest pieces, even in crystal. It's just part of the process, particularly with handcrafted crystal.

Crystal is also softer than regular glass. Dust can scratch your crystal, so washing of your crystal and learning care is essential to keep it in the best shape.

Appropriate maintenance of crystal.

Maintain glassware into contact with your crystal.

Always bring your crystal glasses to break with the foundation facing DOWN, not the fragile rim.

Bring your crystal separately, and do not pile them together!

In case a shard of crystal has broken apart from a glass, you may have the ability to fix it using a sandpaper, made to wash without blemish. Place the crystal glass in direct sunlight to make the epoxy perform its job more efficiently.

Proper washing of crystal.

As previously mentioned, scratches that are noticeable can happen even out of dust. Wash using a cleanser just, wiping lightly with a cloth that does not leave behind any rust.

Do not use goods rimmed crystal, or glasses with engraved gold patterns on the surface! Remember to use the cleansers that are non-irritating.

CHAPTER 25
SUCCESS STORY WITH CRYSTAL HEALING

For many years, many people used crystals in jewelry for the beauty of those. Crystal Healing is regarded as a scientific medicine technique which employs crystals and stones for healing, an ancient practice which dates back to at least 6,000 decades.

The Romans crystals that are used as talismans provide for protection in battle and to promote health. Roman and physicians mixed plant extracts, warmed them and crystals used medicinally.

Ancient Egyptians thought these stones had the power to improve health, and also bury the dead with a quartz crystal, which they thought would direct their loved one safely into the afterlife. Chinese used them to promote healing, enlightenment, and appeal of needs.

And, nowadays, healers, shamans priests use crystals

for their healing properties that are particular. I always had a fascination with crystals and stones but that was as far as it went until I was introduced to crystals and their healing ability at a Mind, Body, & Spirit Festival.

Because crystals vibrate with the power of the planet, they will be able to help you align your body.

With those crystals you also, may vibrate at the energy - Earth Energy! This is where the healing begins.

Pruning yourself in their energy, and with crystals, you are clearing blockages within you which will improve your own all-natural healing abilities.

Our, although most don't realize bodies were designed to be self-correcting and naturally cure themselves.

But as life happens, we sometimes forget to stop and treat ourselves so often, that our bodies escape sync with that healing process, ultimately creating blockages within our physical and mental bodies.

Any blockages in your life force is what causes pains aches, and disease to manifest from the body. It's for this reason, I use crystals daily for strength in a specific area in my own life, for healing that is needed daily, for individual meditation and clarity, or for use in Reiki practice to induce light and love while clearing and cleansing chakras.

Reiki, as just one alternative healing modality, in its translation is Universal Life Force. It is a practice of channeling the universal life energy in a particular pattern to heal and harmonize the mental and physical body and all our Chakras that receives, assimilates, and transmits bodily, emotional, and spiritual energy flowing through our bodies.

There is a clearing technique I use, in addition to a various specific crystal for every chakra to clean blockages that are all in that region.

This clears the way for life force energy to flow for you and through you to maintain the mind, body, and spirit in its divine state of perfect health.

If we maintain our mind, body, and spirit vibrating on a top frequency of love and healing energy, we don't allow aches, pains, and disease to manifest and also settle in the physical body.

Each crystal has its own unique healing property and also a particular Chakra it complies with due.

Our first Chakra, being the Root Chakra, copes with grounding, and largely vibrates together and could be healed using Red, Brown, or Dark Crystals like Red Garnet, Hematite & Black Tourmaline.

The Sacral, Chakra, handling the enjoyment and abdomen facilities, can largely be harmonized with Orange Crystals Carnelian, Amber, and Orange Calcite.

The Third Chakra, being the Solar Plexus Chakra, coping with all the Digestive System and personal power, resonate with and can be treated with Yellow Crystals like Yellow Citrine, and Sunstone.

The Heart chakra, deals with all the Heart, Lungs, and Love. The Heart Chakra vibrates with all Pink or Green crystals like Rose Quartz, Jade, or Green Aventurine at a healing way.

The Throat Chakra, the Chakra, copes with communicating, and resonates with Blue Crystals for example Blue Agate, Sodalite, or Sapphire.

The sixth Chakra knowing and coping with intuition,

vibrates with Violet Crystals like Flourite, & Amethyst, Lolite on a recovery level.

The seventh Chakra, the Crown Chakra, coping with the Central Nervous System & the Divine, resonates best with White or Purple Crystals for example Selenite, Clear Quartz, or Amethyst.

I been using crystals for my healing for a long time, but since starting the use of crystals for healing, I've had some phenomenal success stories, some of which are near and dear to my heart. The first success story is.

From what I am told by many, is. This is definitely an issue with a very long recovery time as he has only gained about three quarters of his motion back in that region without pain thus far in the previous 5 months. Initially, I'd Reiki him we had been sitting and relaxing and also the conclusion of each day.

Then I brought a carnelian chunk to the picture and what he said to me while using the recovery ball was amazing.

The Carnelian ball attracted him amazing warmth, almost like a hot stone everywhere he touched him assisting relax and heal the muscles that had been severed and manipulated during surgery, soothing the pain exactly like a hot stone massage.

The success story is near and dear to me since it has to do with my sister. My sister has Lupus that is basically an autoimmune disorder where your body's immune system attacks its own tissue and organs.

From what I hear and watch her going through, it is a really debilitating disease and physicians just throw different medicines at it as a trial and error thing until they find a drug that works.

Well, she's still in a stage of the disease of not understanding what medication works in assisting every day, the pain that she endures.

I have done Reiki healing numerous instances eased the pain just enough to take off the edge, but it wasn't until I began Crystal Healing Therapy, which she's had relief. I used various distinct Crystals to cleanse and clear her chakras, however I also asked her to wear a Reiki Charged Hematite necklace for a few hours per day. It's been a few weeks and she is reported never having had a really bad pain since.

My third success story in just few weeks has to do with somebody that has degenerative disk disease which is pain in the spine or neck because of a disk in the spine.

Even though there is a somewhat genetic cause to this disease, it caused some kind of trauma or by normal wear and tear to the body.

With this type of disease, there is normally a continuous, usually a baseline pain. It also involves mild to severe episodes of back or neck pain which generally could last anywhere from a few days to a couple months and may be painful during that time, before returning the individual back to what they consider their standard in the pain department.

Rachael was suffering for a long time with degenerative disk disease when she arrived to me. I assisted her with all the healing energy of Reiki along with a carnelian chunk, which I used to treat lower back problems.

After those 2 things, I used Hematite on her that, like

the Belle of the Ball, was for her. As soon as the Hematite stones left contact with skin on her lower back, she noted that a dissolving of this pain almost immediately and stayed for as long as the Hematite stayed on her spine.

I instructed her to continue this practice on her own while she wasn't with me and to wash the Hematite with a Selenite stone to ensure each of the negativity and radicals that the Hematite absorbed from her, could be cleared before returning them to her lower spine.

So despite the therapeutic that is recorded crystal use of many of our ancestors, some discredit the use of these stones.

There aren't a lot of studies to prove or even disprove the power of alternative kinds of medications like crystal healing, acupuncture, Reiki, or even yoga as healing for the mind, body & soul.

This does not mean that those healing practices aren't successful. It merely means that cash isn't being spent on which some consider to be "New Age" recovery; that same healing treatment that's actually curing as old as time.

Also, despite the lack of research for these types of healing procedures, nevertheless about one third of Americans use other kinds of alternative medicine or these. This isn't to say that crystal healing therapy is a cure all.

You should still find the help and medical care from the doctors, however as you can see from these three very different issues and diseases in the above cases, crystal healing stones truly do function to minimize any and all attempts of recovery; whether you've got emotional wounds, specific physical illness, or simply need to increase your energy levels, you may use crystals to vibrate using the same frequencies of earths energy and re-activate your body's own healing capabilities.

CHAPTER 26
CRYSTAL HEALING AND YOUR HEALTH

Crystals have been revered for the beauty and crystal healing effects. From the Melbourne Art Gallery clarify their geological origin and numerous rooms have been allocated to flaunt crystals.

Over time, the art of crystal healing has survived criticism from skeptics so it is somewhat reassuring to see that the science of Geology holds them in such high regard to dedicate rooms in museums to them.

What I want to explain is the possibility exists that crystal recovery may work and endeavor to throw some light on why some people feel such a sense of healing and wellbeing after a crystal healing session.

By means of explanation let's go back to the science laboratory. We learnt that everything is made up of atoms. Solids comprise of lots of moving atoms and look solid since the atoms are so dense (close together) that it looks strong. Dense materials with atoms are those even less dense and liquid are gas.

In fact everything around us, including me and you is composed of those atoms or even smaller particles which are oscillating (moving) however we don't perceive they proceed because our senses cannot pick up that.

Crystals can also be made up of these atoms and oscillate (move) in a specific pace. Studies are done within the past 50 decades or more in UCLA to research this and you can get these on the net.

The way that you move, feel and think etc is unique to you. There's no other person on this world (which you know of so far) that is a duplicate of you.

We become influenced by the vibrations of other people and if you don't believe this simply spend an hour listening to some friend on the telephone that feels down, and by the time they're completed and you put down the phone, you are feeling down also.

We are picking up other people's 'vibes' and enabling individuals to interact with our energy. In precisely the same way the crystals and everything else about us have a vibration that defines a rose quartz crystal by a topaz and so on.

Crystals are distinct in that they have a hierarchical arrangement of the atoms that differs and they oscillate (vibrate) differently making them distinctive from name e.g. smokey quartz differs to amethyst which has an effect when they come into close contact with every one of us.

Our vibration begins to move since the crystal is near us as we would become influenced around us.

This is a portion of the research I referred to earlier and readily available online. It is stated as they interact with our vibrations, that the crystals have a beneficial impact on people, our energy centers and how our personal atoms oscillate alters.

If you consult the books as to the qualities of each crystal there is much information as to how they could affect you and how every crystal can cure different emotions etc..

There is testimony enough for this to matter, that they

170

feel different after they've undergone a crystal recovery.

Whilst some people don't think, there has to be some reason why people feel different. Combine that with all the studies and it becomes open to uncertainty as to if it could be just a placebo effect.

The healer places crystals required on or round the client's body or energy field. The client is usually lying down on a massage mattress or the ground. Ideal conditions are if the room is dim; there are candles along with some soft music or some nice smelling incense.

The notion is that the customer relaxes along with the crystals do their job. The length of time it takes depends on the recovery that is needed.

It's stated that crystals change the method by which the energy centers also known as chakras are vibrating and they undo emotional and energetic blockages in the energy field, and the physical body.

New energy may enter, by unblocking these and it'll flow enhancing life, health and the vitality.

So crystals are a tool for bringing healing and balance to the body, thoughts, emotions and spirit. Whether it is for you or not can be determined out of it and your personal experience might be useful if you could try it on your own.

Don't expect that two healings or only one will work wonders. It has taken you months, sometimes years of neglect of particular regions of your own life and there is no magic wand to whisk it away. That is life, not television and recovery takes time.

Crystal Therapy for Ailments

Crystal therapy is a treatment that is used to give treatment for various ailments like pain and anxiety.

The quick pace lifestyle and working hours have given birth to diseases like stress and body pain. This is a technique which helps a lot in providing comfort. This therapy has been in use since the time immemorial.

In the crystal treatment, crystals and the stones are widely used. It is believed that these crystals help in providing the healing effects on the human body.

Some of the stones and crystals are thought to

possess the curative nature. These stones and crystals are put on the effective role so as to deliver an effect.

This healing treatment is essentially a science. There is no scientific evidence for this therapeutic technique.

But it's commonly utilized in order to provide the comfort effect. These crystals when implemented on the skin, provides a calming effect.

The science behind this healing therapy is that it stimulates the skin cells. Then, this leads to the emission of these enzymes and hormones that help in providing relaxation.

It's believed that the mother character owns cure for various ailments. There are various materials which contain healing properties that are specific.

These crystals are employed to have a healing impact. These crystals are utilized to offer the rejuvenating effect.

The principle of crystal therapy is simple. On the area of the body that is affected by the pain, the stones and crystals are supplied in this.

These work on the energy grids of their body. The crystals are utilized to remove the negative and adverse energy. In providing effect on the 10, these result.

There are experts which are currently offering crystal therapy. Even though it hasn't been proven provide has certain healing impact or not.

However, the use of this therapy reflects its benefits. This treatment has contributed health benefit. We cannot conclude that this treatment doesn't have some advantage.

You can use the crystal therapy to get perfect relief from the pain. The stones and crystals have been put on different parts of the body having effected by the pain. This treatment is very effective in providing comfort.

Stones and the crystals in the form that is heated are placed to provide relaxation. The hidden healing power of the stones helps in taking away the stress and worry. This results in offering a soothing influence on the mind.

One interesting fact connected with crystal treatment is that it doesn't show any side effect. One take this therapy in order to eliminate pain and tension.

174

This is a very effective technique which can reduce pain without supplying any side effect. Crystals and the natural stones will enhance your health standards.

CHAPTER 27
FREQUENTLY ASKED QUESTIONS ABOUT CRYSTALS

I have discovered that certain questions come up time and again.

Crystals are potent, decorative, and fascinating. They have properties and magic powers. They transmit, regulate, generate, store, and change energy. A quartz crystal can control a radio or watch while crystal lasers are now being used in operation.

Crystals harmonize your entire body, or the air. By taking in energy, they provide protection, and cleansing your air and the surroundings. Many crystals, for example Amazonite, or Black Tourmaline have a construction which absorbs energy.

This means that crystals holds detrimental energies like negative ideas or electromagnetic 'smog', and counteracts the harmful impact. Crystals are also programmed to radiate vibes into the environment, which makes them perfect for enhancing your home or workplace.

They could attract prosperity, friendship love and anything you can imagine into your life. The ability of crystals to focus energy means they may be used for specific tasks, like directing healing energy into a point on the human body or into a psychological blockage.

Crystals divine the future and much more. You can change your life, by harnessing the unique splendor of crystals.

They can bring everything to you your heart needs - if you understand how to get their electricity. Crystals are used for healing.

Healing, in this regard, doesn't mean to make better', it means to make you feel good, improve well-being. In ancient and medieval times, crystals were actually grounded and administered as medicines.

Have our ancestors Now, crystals are used?

Absolutely, crystals have been used for adornment but also for curing not only for thousands of years and to influence life's course. Ancient peoples believed crystals were presents from the gods and that they really carried the essence of a goddess or god. Amber beads have been discovered for example, over 8000 years old, now and amber is employed as a protective stone.

Their charming properties have been recognized in each culture and have been used by magicians, shamans, healers, and astrologers so there is a huge tradition behind their usage these days.

Crystals come in all shapes and sizes. Some are shining, glamorous - and pricey. Others are pieces, seemingly dull until you understand their secrets. Ruby or a diamond could be overlooked in its uncooked state.

Many stones are cut in their normal form, although faceted to enhance their physical appearance. That means you allow it to do its work and can slide a crystal or under your pillow.

For a crystal to perform its magic, it must be magnetized to your energies. This contrasts the crystal to your own objective. It helps to ensure that the crystal will carry out its task and helps focus upon what you want your crystal.

Dedicating a crystal considerably enhances the potency of the crystal clear and ensures good comes out of its use. Wash your crystal under running water to cleanse its energies, then hold it in the hands and position it to respond to you by devoting it to a specific purpose.

Love radiates out from many stones and crystals can be erotic like Red Jasper or powerfully intimate as in the case of Rose Quartz.

A soul mate is attracted by them into an existing relationship. Crystals makes you more open to love and also changes how you feel about yourself.

You can feel like radiating out from several crystals and diamonds, worn over the heart, such stones can be quite soothing.

They've a gentle energy that gives you the capability love and to accept yourself - a necessity to being loved by somebody else. Among the most entertaining ways to experience crystal love is to take a bath.

Pick qualities you search: romance, passion, self-love, recovery for your heart. Clean the crystal and place it inside the water, in which you can add several drops of rose oil. Have a hot soak cloth and absorb the energies. If you share your bath. Beneath your pillow to reinforce its effects, slip the stone at night.

The crystal that appeals to you is the right choice. It is not necessary that a crystal has to be rare or expensive to be effective.

When it comes to crystal power appearance and size matter little. Don't be fooled by shiny bright and large gemstones. These aren't necessarily the best.

Small, crystals that are attractive have exactly the identical energy - and cost a fantastic deal less. Notice that crystal catches your eye, when you visit a crystal store.

It is going to most likely be the one for you. If you are looking for a specific crystal, dip your hands and the one which sticks to your hand has your name on it.

Bear in mind that everybody is different. We radiate different frequencies, we have different perspectives, different family patterns. So there is no 1 magic 'cure all' crystals.

What works for you will not necessarily work for your friend, but there'll be a different one that does. So don't be scared to experiment crystals rather than following what somebody else tells you is the way to do it

There is an emotional or spiritual condition that is manifested to draw your attention to. Crystals gently handle these underlying conditions and bring you back into holistic equilibrium which is the real th definition of recovery I prefer.

One important thing is that crystals do also absorb negative energies so they require regular cleaning differently or else they quit working. Put them out in the sun to recharge and then hold them under running water for few minutes.

They may also be placed into salt or brown rice overnight or put on a sizable quartz bunch or carnelian to wash and re-energize.

CONCLUSION

Crystal healing is the use of crystals to cause favorable and healing changes in body the mind, and spirit. For me, crystals energized me have cured illness, cured emotional trauma, assisted me to conquer dependence, and changed my life!

All gemstones carry their own vibrational frequencies and by putting them on your own body or you can alter your vibrational frequency.

Crystals act as amplifiers. They bring about the desired outcome that much faster and enhance your intention.

There are many crystals for addressing physical and psychological issues out there in most shaped, sizes, and colors and they each have their own properties.

However, you locate the crystals that you think you want and can drive yourself crazy trying to study.

You should really do it the manner that is opposite, the crystal selections on you!

So, if you're in a crystal store choosing crystals out to take home with you, simply stop and go back which you touched because most probably that was.

After You Buy your new natural treasures there are. I'm sure you are most likely excited and want to use them already, but these steps are a part of the crystal healing procedure. You will need to cleanse your crystals of any energy it has consumed.

You will also have to cleanse your crystals from time to time based on how you utilize them. There are numerous effective methods for clearing crystals.

Among the best ways and the simplest is to set them on your hands, holding the intention to clean all negative energy and hold it.

The faucet functions. Some methods for clearing are to set them or bury them in the ground for a day or more, or by simply utilizing your breath.

Step two is also to set the intention it will be used to your higher good or the good of anyone else that uses it and to attune your crystal to your frequency.

All you need to do would be to hold the crystal in

your hands, close your eyes, and then set these two intentions.

You may say them or simply think them, either way is effective. Step three would be to charge your crystals. Place your crystals in direct sun for a minimum of 5 hours.

You can also place them overnight beneath the light of a new or full moon. For what you're likely to be using them, the last step is to program your crystals.

For example it is possible to say that they should be utilized for general recovery purposes, or for security, or grounding, etc.. .

This may not be accomplished. The reason that one can do this step is since programming a crystal for a particular use farther attunes it to the vibration of your needs; bringing about the desired outcome even faster.

To perform this crystal in your hands and say aloud (not in your head)"This crystal is going to be used for ___", and fill in the blank. Repeat those words 3 to 4 times to program the crystal clear. Now you're ready to utilize your crystals that are new!

There are many ways you can use your crystals; it all depends on your needs. Here are just a couple of ways in which you are able to use your precious gemstones:

You can wear them as jewelry or carry one or two beside you in your pocket or handbag (in case you employ them in such a manner, do not forget you have to cleanse your crystals more frequently because they will more readily liven up any negativity at the surroundings that you're in).

You can also meditate with your by placing them on crystals or about you, which will greatly amplify your meditation.

You can clear and balance your chakras using crystals by putting corresponding stones and intending to clean and balance them.

You can keep crystals inside the room or on your workspace for draining or protection. You can place at night to improve and remember your dreams under your pillow, or for sleep.

The possibilities are infinite with crystals and they're sure to enhance your life!

I hope that you enjoy using crystals!

Best wishes.